EARLY BOOK REVIEWS

"In her memoir, Cancer Don't Care, Michelle Sandlin shares her personal battle with a cancer diagnosis. With unflinching honesty and surprising humor, Michelle describes each fear, doubt, and triumph in navigating the path to save her life. This book would benefit anyone with an overwhelming diagnosis or someone who loves them."

- Cheryl Howe, Author

"Cancer Don't Care is one woman's intimate, courageous, gut wrenching, and heartwarming account of her own personal breast cancer journey. An insider's guide to everything you need to know if you've been diagnosed with breast cacer, this book offers life lessons that are relevant for all of us. It's a story of loss, love, letting go, and rebirth. From the first page to the last, I was in awe, engaged, and inspired. Thank you, Michelle, for taking us with you on this life changing and affirming journey."

- Ann Gladstone

"Michelle's story affected me deeply and moved me to compassion. From her needing the perfect cancer binder, to using her beloved late mother's Sharpies to take notes, to desiring the just-right wig…I found myself relating to her on many levels. Perhaps it's because she's an original Louisiana girl like me, or maybe it's because we're both writers. Regardless, I love Michelle's message to keep moving, stay the course, and know that there is life after cancer."

– Cathey Nickell,
Children's Book Author and School Speaker

CANCER DON'T CARE

A Memoir

Michelle Sandlin

For my husband Kenny, for being my rock and my support animal throughout my journey and our life together.

For my daughter Kendall, for paving my journey with love, laughter, devotion, and strength.

For my brother Michael, for the promise of always being there for each other.

And though she be but little, she is fierce.
- William Shakespeare
(A Midsummer Night's Dream)

TABLE OF CONTENTS

FOREWORD
BY: KENDALL SANDLIN

As soon as my mom told me she was diagnosed with breast cancer, I broke down. You never expect for someone close to you to ever become sick in such a serious way, and so I was scared. My mom immediately told me to stop and said we were not going to cry or be sad about this. She went on to tell me she was going to beat this, and that she wasn't going to allow any sadness, only positivity. That brought me so much comfort, and completely changed my outlook about her diagnosis, because I knew she was going to beat this.

Right away, I began to try to comfort my mom and let her know I would be there for her through everything. I offered as much positivity and support as I could, whether it was going to appointments with her, bringing my sons to spend time with her, or just laughing on the phone with her to brighten up her day.

During my mom's cancer journey, I also ended up having a genetic test after we learned that she was a carrier for the BRCA1 gene mutation. I wanted to find out if I had the mutation as well, and it turns out that I do. This means that I am also at high risk for developing breast cancer. So, I immediately thought about how that would affect my life moving forward, and more importantly, the life of my three children. After advisement from my doctors, my mom, and the understanding of how it would significantly reduce my own breast cancer risk, I made the decision to have a double mastectomy. Watching my mom power through breast cancer the way she did, let me know deep in my soul that I could do the same, and I HAD to do the same through my preventative care.

I was there for my mom throughout her journey, and now she is here for me. She has brought me so much strength, and I admire her so much for coming out on top since the day of her diagnosis. I aspire to be like her and to be able to comfort my children in the same way that she has continued to comfort me.

FOREWORD
BY: CANDY ARENTZ, MD, MBA, FACS
Breast Surgical Oncology

Being diagnosed with breast cancer is hard. We all know someone who has been treated with this disease, but until it happens to you, it all seems very far off. As a breast cancer surgeon, I tell women (and an occasional man) that they have been diagnosed with breast cancer every day. This is the worst part of my job. However, it is also the day that I can give hope and start devising a plan to overcome the disease.

On the first visit, I invite all family members and friends to join in the appointment. If some are not available in person, they are welcome to join virtually. It is important that everyone hear the treatment plan because the breast cancer patient cannot understand the depth and complexity alone.

I remember Michelle's first appointment with me following her diagnosis. Both her husband and her brother came with her. She later remarked to me that most of the details we discussed that day were hard to comprehend, as she was still in shock from the diagnosis, and was just doing her best to digest all of this new information. I often have people tell me later that our first meeting was just a blur and sometimes they do not even recognize me at our second appointment because they were so overwhelmed. My goal is to provide my patients with a plan, so that's what I did with Michelle at our first meeting, which helps take away some of the fear of the unknown. The fear of the unknown is 75 percent of the problem, but we are all stronger than we think.

The emotional well-being of the patient, family, and friends is key to surviving breast cancer. I also believe that maintaining positivity and productivity in your life after the diagnosis of breast cancer improves health and well-being. This is something that Michelle and I discussed throughout her treatment. From the very beginning, she stated her desire to stay as active as possible, while maintaining her positive attitude. Breast cancer patients need someone to talk to, cry on, and laugh with just as they did prior to being diagnosed. Be present. Be kind. Be available.

The best part of my job is telling patients, like Michelle, that they are cancer-free! After the hard-fought battle with breast cancer, the relief and happy tears at the end mean the most. Michelle has told me many times since I was able to deliver the good news to her, just what an emotional release that moment was for her. I am thankful every day for these appointments.

PREFACE

Introspection

This is not the book I ever thought I'd be writing. But here we are.

It was born out of a place of quiet contemplation. It's a place I have frequented most of my life. Even as a small child, I was easily swept away in my own thoughts. A million miles away. Analyzing everything. Examining my life at every stage — my childhood, my choices, my relationships, my passions, my career — always trying to figure things out.

The more perplexing thoughts often drift out of my head and through my fingertips onto the waiting page. It's how I express myself, but it's also how I reach important decisions and conclusions about the world within me, as well as the world around me. It's where the emotional rubber meets the road.

Introspection is such a valuable tool because of what it forces us to do — to take a closer look at our current situation, reflect on how we got there, stare down life's biggest challenges, and find answers to our greatest questions.

What This Book Is

This book is my way of processing my thoughts, feelings, and insights about what happened, what I went through, and what it's like to be on the other side. It's about overcoming adversity by channeling your inner strength, maintaining a positive attitude, requiring the same of those around you, and fighting your way through. It's about self-motivation, acceptance, and inspiration on the road to healing and inner peace.

I certainly don't have all the answers, but I learned some valuable lessons about myself, others, love, faith, attitude, and so much more along the way.

Like most things, I needed to write it all down, look at it

through a microscope, dissect it, and assign my own meaning. That has enabled me to gain some perspective about my experience, how it changed me, and how it might help others too.

My Promise to You

One of the promises I made to myself, and I make to you, is to write this without self-censoring. I won't sugarcoat my feelings, physical shortcomings, or raw emotions. I'm handing it off to you the same way it happened — like an unfiltered selfie. There isn't a more authentic way to share my experience. That's how it has the best shot of helping and encouraging you or someone you love.

My hope is that this book will be a source of inspiration you can grab whenever you need it. Whenever you need some reassurance. Whenever you need some hope. And especially, whenever you feel alone.

On Writing This Book

I was lost in my own thoughts. I had been for a few months. Struggling to process my breast cancer experience. I knew I needed to take a deep dive into my experience from this safe distance I like to call the other side. To see it from a healthy angle, in hopes of gaining some valuable insight about myself and my journey. And to use my experience as a way of helping others.

Then one day, I posted a video on my Facebook page about how I was grappling with everything that had happened, and trying to figure out what my life looks like after cancer.

The message of my video was: *What the hell was that? To find out, I've decided to write a book. A book I'd been unknowingly writing since the day I was diagnosed.*

It's true. I had been writing this book all along. It was everywhere. Bits and pieces were written in my journals, in notebooks, on index cards, and digitally recorded in Apple Notes on my iPhone. There were videos, photos, and social media posts. In some form or another, I had documented my entire journey. Now I needed to go back, revisit, ruminate, reflect, and remember.

Right after I posted the video, I began to feel the excitement rise within me. I was committed, and I didn't want to waste another minute. *Let's do this.*

All my juices started flowing, and before I knew it, I was holding a lime green Post-it notes pad in one hand, and a black Sharpie marker in the other. This activity required a bold, bright color, and I deliberately chose lime green because it reminded me of my mom. And I chose the Sharpie because Sharpies are decisive and permanent. Once you write something with a Sharpie, there's no going back; it's forever.

So, as fast as my hand could write, I began jotting down themes and ideas. Frantically writing on the lime green squares of paper, tearing off each sheet from the pad, and moving on to the next. Attaching each note to the surface of my desk in random fashion. In no time it became a sea of lime green. It looked chaotic, yet beautiful. It was my story, and it was ready to be written.

And so it begins….

INTRODUCTION

Everyone seems to refer to their breast cancer experience as a journey, and it definitely is that. I've thought a lot about what to call mine. In keeping with the positive attitude that I fought hard to maintain throughout my battle, perhaps it was more of an adventure. But I would be lying if I didn't say it was also a storm. And some storms leave a path of destruction in their wake. Some things are demolished or lost, while others must be rebuilt, repaved, and reconstructed. But, through it all, I kept reminding myself that all storms eventually pass, and sometimes things can change and improve really fast, even after the worst of storms. Grey clouds lift and are replaced by blue skies, birds begin to tweet, and all feels calm and *normal* again.

Where to Begin?

It's hard to know where this story begins. There was no break in the action between losing my mom, the crippling grief that followed, getting *healthy,* the pandemic, and finding a lump in my right breast. It all runs together.

When my mom died in March of 2019, my entire world came crashing down. It left me yearning for a new sense of gravity. A way to feel my feet on solid ground. Instead, I was forced to step over all the shattered pieces that my mom's death left behind. To search for answers beneath the rubble. But her death was sudden and unexpected, leaving me with as many questions as answers, not just about her life, but my own.

My North Star was gone, and I was lost. And I could feel myself spiraling in a way that threatened to take me under. I knew I had to yank myself up before it was too late. So, I picked up a red pen and began editing my own story. Rewriting my life. Determined to change the ending.

It started with the simple realization that the only two things I can really control are what I eat and drink, and how much I move my body. That's when I decided to make some significant lifestyle changes. I knew it wouldn't take the grief away, but it would at least provide a positive diversion. So, I bought a Peloton bike and prepared to pedal my way into a healthy routine, while letting go of some of my physical and emotional baggage that was weighing me down.

Two weeks later my Peloton arrived, and after the first ride, I was hooked. I began eating a healthy diet, I stopped drinking alcohol, and I dropped a few pounds. Soon, working out became an obsession. A way to flush out my system. To sweat away my grief. And to let the toxins hit the floor below me.

Before long, I was working out one to two hours a day, six days a week. I looked great. I felt great, and I was in the best shape of my life. For two years, I dedicated myself to this new and improved way of life, consistently pushing and challenging myself. But sometimes your whole world ruptures. Not once, but twice. Each time without warning.

That's when God said, "Wait, there's more. Now you have breast cancer."

That's right. You can be living your healthiest, cleanest life ever. But guess what? Cancer don't care. It literally gives zero fucks.

My mom taught me and my brother to be scared of damn near everything. She was a chronic worrier, mostly about things that never even happen. She said it kept her awake at night. But fear about this thing that actually did happen, somehow never made it onto her list of worries. *Cancer. How did she miss that one?*

Nonetheless, there I was, standing at the base of a mountain that I never thought I would have to climb. *Do I even have the right shoes or equipment? I will have to find out as I go.* Putting one foot above the other, I began my ascent.

CHAPTER 1: HOW IT STARTED

Life is full of unexpected, unscripted moments that you never thought would happen to you, but here we are.

Foreshadowing

Signs were everywhere. Shouting at me. Trying to get my attention. My anxiety was like a runaway train, and I was having trouble concentrating. Just like before. Just like the week my mom died. Something big was coming. I could feel it. There was this sense of foreboding, but I kept ignoring it. The more it nagged at me, the more I said *go away*.

But it was obvious, the wind had begun to blow in a different direction. One I never saw coming. Something was wrong, but the timing didn't make sense. Now? After all the work I'd done to get healthy and make myself at least semi-whole again after losing my mom? I was so close to getting my life back together. How was everything about to come crashing down? Again, and so soon? It must be a mistake. That's why I ignored it. That's why I pushed it away.

It's easy to look back now and see the warning signs. Something was bubbling in the background. The foreshadowing words in my journal that read: *My life feels like it has fallen apart and been put back together incorrectly. Something feels off, but I just can't put my finger on it. All I know is that it's time for me to get my life together.*

Little did I know, the opposite was about to happen. My whole life was about to fall apart — for the second time in two years — and would never be the same. Parts of me would be removed, relocated, and reconstructed. Like deleting the bad verses of my story. Only I didn't control the narrative. *Did I ever really control the narrative?*

The two weeks leading up to my diagnosis were chaotic and overwhelming. Much like the week leading up to my mom's death. And I was creatively blocked, just like before. An unmistakable, strange parallel. And now there I was again, struggling to get everything done. My plate was so full I could hardly lift it. Both times I kept thinking that something's got to give.

But this time was different. This time all the healthy changes I'd made to my lifestyle weren't enough to prevent the inevitable. It was as if everything was conspiring against me. In spite of how good I thought I looked on the outside, there was a relentless poison growing on the inside. And I was oblivious to the power it had over me, and the damage it had already done. I didn't even know it was there.

Some years ago, I wrote the words: *When your life turns upside down, you have to create a new sense of gravity.* So often it happens that words and phrases and poetry just come out of nowhere and land on me like a fly. I try not to question it. I just write it down, like the dutiful scribe that I am. It's not uncommon for years to pass before the meaning finally reveals itself. Then I understand.

Lies We Tell Ourselves

I was having a sharp, shooting pain in my right breast. It was intermittent, so it took me a while to acknowledge it. As quickly as it would show up, it would leave. So, I kept dismissing it. Not ignoring it, but dismissing it and mischaracterizing it as a potential side effect of the COVID-19 vaccine. I may have had some swelling too, but mostly there was just some tenderness.

My second vaccine was just a few days ago, so that's probably it. That wasn't it. *Maybe I pulled a muscle while lifting weights, or maybe I needed to wear a more supportive sports bra.* That wasn't it either. I thought there must be a simple explanation, especially since I'd had my annual mammogram four and a half months earlier, and the results had been all clear. There was no reason for me to jump to cancer. It was the last thing on my mind. So, I downplayed it. But I guess that's the way things happen; we just dismiss until we can't dismiss anymore.

Nonetheless, I decided to alert my OBGYN's office by sending a message through the online patient portal.

I have been having some breast pain (right breast) over the last few weeks immediately following my second COVID-19 vaccine. It doesn't seem to be going away, so I wanted to let you know and ask what I should do. I had the vaccines on April 2nd and 23rd.

Within minutes, I received a response from one of the nurses.

Good afternoon Michelle, it is not uncommon for women to experience breast tenderness due to the COVID-19 vaccine. It may cause swelling of the lymph nodes. It is the reason we encourage women to wait 3-6 months to have a mammogram after receiving the vaccine. If you feel it is necessary to be seen, please call the office to schedule an appointment. If you have any other questions, please don't hesitate to call me, or send another message.

The nurse didn't seem alarmed, which made me feel better. So, I carried on. Still, I was struggling to get things done. I had taken almost no time off in a year, and I needed a breather. I wanted to think, review what I was doing, re-prioritize, and move towards something meaningful. I needed a goal, but there wasn't one in sight. I was stuck somewhere in between my grief and trying to figure out what was next in my life. I needed a little space just for me, but I didn't know how to make that happen. The moment felt all wrong. In hindsight, you'd think I would have recognized that moment. The one just before the storm makes landfall, but it wasn't even in the forecast. It could not have been more quiet. Yes, it was hectic, but strangely calm.

A few days went by. Then a few more days went by. After a couple of weeks, I was still having the pain. It just kept popping up, mostly when I was in bed at night. It was the only time I was still and quiet enough to notice. The pain was becoming more frequent, and the intensity was increasing. It felt like someone was poking my right breast with a needle. I had reached a point where the pain was vying for my full attention.

That's when I found it.

It was late, and I couldn't sleep. The pain was persistent. So, I started moving my fingers around the area where I felt the pain. Instantly I felt something I had never felt before. *Is that a lump? Is it? How can I be sure? Is that a lump?*

The more I felt it, the more surreal the moment became. I kept touching it over and over again. Removing my hand, then touching the area again as if for the first time. My husband Kenny was asleep next to me, and I didn't want to wake him. I didn't want to alarm him. Not yet.

So, I gently sat up in bed and felt the area again. It was small, but I could feel it. Almost like a small pebble under my skin. *Where did this come from?* I laid back down and felt it again, comparing the same area in my other breast. I sat up again. Checked my left breast, then my right. Again and again. Then I stopped abruptly because I was freaking myself out. I wasn't ready to acknowledge this, whatever *this* was. It would have to wait until morning.

When I woke up the next day, Kenny was already downstairs feeding the dogs. So, alone in my bathroom, I walked over to the mirror, lifted my shirt, and felt my breasts again. It was not my imagination. There was something there. *Is it just some swelling, or something worse?* I slowly lifted my arms up and back down. Felt one breast, then the other. *What is this? I think it's a fucking lump.*

That was the moment. I had to give in and stop battling all the voices in my head. I knew what I knew, and it was a lump. Yes, a lump, and it had my full, undivided attention. The red flags could stop waving now.

. . .

I went downstairs to find Kenny. I needed him to feel it too.

"Remember that pain I've been having in my right breast? Well, I think I can feel a lump. I want to see if you can feel it."

I took his hand and placed it over the area of my breast where I felt the lump.

"Well, do you feel it?"

He gave a half chuckle and said, "The only thing I feel is a boob."

"No, no, no. It's right here. I know you can feel it?"

"Nope. It must not be that big. Are you sure there's a lump?"

"Yes, I'm positive."

Repeatedly, I took his hand and put it right over the lump, and repeatedly he told me that he didn't feel anything. Looking back, I am not sure if he really couldn't feel anything, or whether he was in denial – same as me – and couldn't believe his own fingers. Telling him I found a lump on my breast was way outside the realm of anything close to normal. So, no matter how many times I took his hand and insisted that he feel it again, he gave me the same answer, "Just a boob."

While that should have been reassuring, it wasn't. I could feel the lump. There was no mistaking it for anything else. It was unlike anything I had ever felt before. I knew it wasn't right. I knew it was a lump. And I knew I had to make an appointment to see my doctor.

Looking back, I can't believe I waited so long to make the call, except that those were strange, unprecedented times due to the pandemic. Still, I should have known better. I had never experienced breast pain like that before, and this was my first lump. I'm not even sure when the lump appeared. All I know is that the pain led to my self-examination, which allowed me to find the lump. And when I did, I had a hard time admitting that it was a lump, even to myself. I tried to talk myself out of it. *It's swelling, not a lump. No! It's a lump.*

Being Your Own Advocate

You would think that calling the doctor's office to say you found a lump in your breast would be met with urgency. Much to my surprise, it wasn't. It was more like calling to schedule a routine dental appointment.

"Hello, I sent a message through the online patient portal a few weeks ago describing a pain I've been having in my right breast. Well, I now seem to have a lump there too and need to see the doctor right away. What does he have available this week?"

"Unfortunately, the first available appointment is three weeks from Thursday at 11 a.m. Shall I put you down?"

That was the first shot in the battle. I felt rage rising throughout my whole body. Writhing. Surging. I had already decided I needed to see the doctor pronto, so waiting three weeks for an appointment was unacceptable.

I felt the panic deep in my chest as I took a deep breath and steadied my tone.

"No, you can't put me down for three weeks from now. I have just discovered a lump in my breast, and I need to see the doctor ASAP."

"I'm sorry, but he is completely booked for the next three weeks."

"Well, that's not going to work. This is urgent, and I need to see him this week, otherwise, I will need to schedule an appointment with one of the other doctors in the practice who can see me this week. I'm sorry, but this can't wait."

"Can I put you on a brief hold?"

"Yes."

I guess that got her attention, because about a minute later, she came back on the line.

"How about tomorrow at 9 a.m.?"

"Perfect! I will be there."

My assumption had been wrong. I thought as soon as I said the words: *lump in my right breast* to the person on the other end of the phone, that the Red Sea would part, and I would be ushered into the doctor's office the very next day. I am still surprised by the lackadaisical response to my frantic tone. *Couldn't she hear the fear in my voice? What about lump didn't she understand?*

In many ways, this episode set the tone for how things were

going to go in terms of navigating the frustrating waters of the healthcare system. It taught me the importance of being your own advocate. Nobody is going to fight your way in for you like *you*. You might be told that there aren't any appointments available at this time, or that you can't be seen for a few weeks. That's unacceptable. Be persistent and assertive. Keep making calls. Explain your situation as many times as you need to, and eventually you will get it done. And never – I mean never – take no for an answer.

Here's My Personal Cell Phone Number

Fortunately, the doctor's appointment was first thing in the morning, so I didn't have to sweat it out all day. Kenny went with me. It was the first time he had attended a doctor's appointment with me in years. So, he'd never met this doctor until the moment after we heard that knock on the door.

"Hey Doc! This is my husband, Ken."

"Nice to meet you, Ken. I'm a little surprised to see your wife again so soon. I know I just saw her a few months ago."

"Yes, in January," I said.

"Right, so what's going on?"

"I've been having some pain in my right breast, and now there's a small lump. I initially thought it might be related to my COVID-19 vaccine, but…"

"I understand. It looks like you had a mammogram a little over four months ago and the result was normal, but let's take a look and see what's going on. Please lie straight back and place your hands under your head."

My hands felt sweaty as they touched each other underneath my head.

"I feel what you feel. Right there at eleven o'clock. There does seem to be a mass there, but I don't think it's cancer. We do need to find out what it is though, so I want you to have another mammogram and an ultrasound ASAP. I am putting the order in right now, so you can call and get it scheduled as soon as you leave here."

"Mass? I don't like that word."

"The fact is that there is something there. We just don't know what it is yet. That's why I want you to have another mammogram and an ultrasound. Go ahead and get dressed and let's visit in my office."

After I got dressed, we went into the doctor's private office to talk. As we sat down, I looked over at Kenny, and he looked a little concerned. I didn't want him to be. Not yet anyway. Then I looked at the doctor. I tried, but I couldn't read him. I didn't get the impression that he thought there was anything to worry about. Not until he pulled out a yellow sticky note and began scribbling.

"This is my personal cell phone number. I am going out of town for a few days, but call me if…"

I don't even know how that sentence ended. I just knew I'd been given a doctor's personal cell phone number, which never happens. *So, this might be serious.* Still, I was not thinking it was cancer. I just assumed that if the doctor thought it was cancer, he would have come right out and said it. He didn't, and I was holding on to that, along with the sticky note.

Side of the Road

The moment we cleared the parking garage, I began placing calls. The first one was to the Breast Care Center at the hospital to schedule my mammogram and ultrasound. The same place where I'd had the normal mammogram four and a half months earlier.

The call wasn't going well. After a series of basic questions — name, date of birth, insurance, name of referring physician — I was placed on hold. The hold time was getting longer, so I pulled my car over and parked on a nearby residential street. My nerves were already rattled, and I could feel my blood starting to boil.

The appointment scheduler came back on the line only to tell me there were no appointments available at either of her two locations for the next three weeks. *Nope!* I insisted that I needed to have this done tomorrow, and she insisted that there were no openings.

She then gave me the phone numbers of all the other satellite locations in the Houston area. For once, I was glad to live in a city known for its sprawling healthcare community.

Frantically, I called each location as fast as Kenny called out their phone numbers.

"Hi, I need to schedule a mammogram and ultrasound for some time in the next few days."

"Sorry, but we don't have anything available for the next several weeks."

"Hi, I need to schedule a mammogram and ultrasound for some time in the next few days."

"Sorry, but we don't have anything available…"

I hit brick wall after brick wall. Same story, different location.

While I was trying to work some miracle on my phone, Kenny was on his phone trying to find an opening at any of the locations through the online scheduling app. With each call, I begged a little more. *Please, are you sure you can't squeeze me in?*

Frustrated, I placed one more call. It was to the last location on the list. Then a miracle did happen. As I was on hold with the appointment scheduler, I received another incoming call. I recognized the phone number as belonging to one of the locations that had already turned me away. So, I quickly switched over to the incoming call.

"Hello?"

"Hi Mrs. Sandlin. We just spoke. You had called about scheduling your mammogram and ultrasound for this week. Well, I have great news. We've just had a cancellation for tomorrow."

Boom shakalaka!

The Breast Care Center

I was grumpy on the drive over to the Breast Care Center. I'm always grumpy when I am anxious and nervous, and I was definitely anxious and nervous.

We walked in, and Kenny sat down while I checked myself in. The receptionist handed me a clipboard with the required paperwork, and I hurried to fill everything out. I don't remember waiting very long, and I barely even remember the mammogram.

What I remember is the ultrasound. It was performed by a nurse who had a welcoming smile that said *don't worry*.

The room was cold, and the lighting was low. I did my best to stay still as she rubbed the jelly-covered wand around my right breast. Over and over the same spot. The wand was sticky as it rolled across my skin. This all seemed fairly routine, until it didn't. I just watched her face. Her expression. Looking for something that would reassure me. There was nothing discernable as she continued to push the wand. It was uncomfortable and seemed to last forever.

"Are you almost done?"

"Just a few more minutes."

"Are you able to tell me if you can see anything?"

"No, the radiologist will come in and talk to you when I'm done."

. . .

Right on cue, the radiologist walked in. Her face was long and serious as she studied the ultrasound images. My eyes were fixed on her eyes. I felt the tension grow as I watched her expression. It was written all over her face. Something was wrong.

"Is something wrong? Do you see something?"

"Yes, I do see something."

"What do you think it is? Please tell me the truth."

"I think it might be positive."

"Positive? What does that mean?"

"Positive for cancer. I think it's cancer."

That's when all of my words started spewing out uncontrollably. The first one out the door was, *fuck,* followed by, *I'm sorry.* So much anger was balling up inside me so quickly. My voice cracked, and my eyes burned, but no tears. I was too shocked to cry. On the verge of a panic attack. I couldn't breathe.

My chest was tightening. I was talking fast and breathing heavy. I went on and on about my healthy lifestyle and my mom's death and how none of this made sense.

The radiologist was careful not to confirm anything.

"How sure are you?" I asked.

"I'm about 80 percent sure it's cancer."

"Holy shit! So you're only 20 percent sure it's not cancer? I'm no mathematician, but those are terrible odds."

"I know, but we can't be sure until we do a biopsy, and I'd like you to have one as soon as possible. We need to reach out to your doctor first, but I'd like to do the biopsy today. Could you be back here in two hours?"

"Wow. That sounds urgent. Yes. Of course."

My heart was racing, and my body was shaking as I rushed to get dressed. Then I walked out to the waiting area to find Kenny.

"Come on. We have to go. Right now. I have to be back here in two hours for a biopsy."

He looked confused and said, "OK."

I walked as fast as I could out of the building, into the parking lot, and headed straight for the car. Kenny was several paces behind me, struggling to keep up. All I wanted was to get in the car and get out of there. It was taking too long, so I circled back to where Kenny was and quietly said over my right shoulder, "They think it's cancer."

"Oh my God! Really?"

"Yes. Come on, and I will fill you in after we get in the car."

The two hours gave us just enough time to run home, walk the dogs, choke down a couple of protein bars, and for me to make the dreaded phone call to my brother Michael.

Since losing my mom, my relationship with Michael had reached a whole new level. We are each other's first and last call of the day, as well as countless others in between. And I wouldn't want it any other way. There were so many unspoken promises between us. We had a shared past, present, and future. A shared childhood. A shared bathroom growing up. My longest living relationship with another human being. He has been in my life now longer than my mom. Longer than any other. Like twins, we feel each other's pain. We worry, like Mom worried. We're hardwired that way. We're supposed to lift each other up and be the voice of Mom when it's the one voice we long to hear the most.

So, Michael knew about the pain, the lump, the doctor's appointment, the mammogram, the ultrasound, and he was now waiting for me to call him and let him know that everything was fine. Everything wasn't fine, and I knew this latest development would be almost more than he could handle. I took a breath, made the call, and he picked up on the first ring.

"How did it go?"

"Well, it's kind of still going. We are at the house for a quick bite and to walk the dogs, but they want me to come back this afternoon for a biopsy."

"Oh geez. A biopsy?"

"Yep, they saw something on the ultrasound, and they think it could be cancer."

"What? Are you kidding?"

"I wish I was, but the radiologist looked serious when she was reading the results of my ultrasound. She said she thinks it might be cancer, so I need to have a biopsy right away to know for sure. Anyway, we're not going to worry until it's time to worry. Please just think positive thoughts, and I will call you when we get back home."

. . .

Kenny and I returned for the biopsy right on schedule. Within moments the nurse called my name. It was the same one from earlier. As I climbed onto the hospital bed, I asked her if she would hold my hand. She smiled and took my hand and never let it go until the biopsy was completed. I felt scared and lonely lying there, turned slightly onto my left side. I kept my eyes closed and grimaced with each tug as the radiologist performed the biopsy.

When it was over, I was given a heart-shaped breast pillow as my parting gift. And the radiologist told me she would call me with the results Monday or Tuesday. It was only Friday.

So, we wait.

Bargaining with God

As I waited, not so patiently, for the results of my biopsy (AKA: my diagnosis), I began secretly bargaining with God. It's what you do.

Journal: June 20, 2021

This one is for God…

Please don't let me have cancer. I've already been through too much over the last two years. My life shouldn't be turned upside down again and some more. I need a break. And yes, I know I haven't exactly been connecting with You and my religion much since my mom's death, but it's been too hard. Or I've been too doubtful or something…So now, today, I ask You for the strength to heal and reconnect with my faith and the Jewish life I've always led. Faith in God. Belief in God. Belief that You are representative of all things good and will show me the way. I must put my hands in Your hands. Clearly, I have no control, and whatever choices I have made to live clean and healthy were somehow not enough. Please lead me. Please be there for me. Please give me strength through Your strength. I am asking for Your help. My mom's not here and I need her more than ever. She would be so upset at the shear possibility that I could have cancer. I've been trying to figure out what she would say to me in this moment, but I am at a loss. I know she would be scared, same as me. And I am indeed scared.

I don't know how to deal with this constant feeling of being out of control. When did I give up control? The answer is that I didn't. It was stripped from me without my permission as I slept during the early hours of March 28, 2019. My innocence was stripped from me that day too, as life as I knew it quickly began to unravel and come apart at the seams. Every element of my life changed in a flash. And as I drove to the hospital, I spoke to You then. I prayed and I screamed at the top of my lungs, "please don't take my mom."

But You did take her, and I'm still angry at you for that. But this new thing now, seems like a dirty joke. And so, I have to ask You and beg You, please don't let me have cancer. Let's bargain. I will do something else instead. My life is in Your hands, and I have every belief that this is not meant to happen to me. Please just spare me. Please God, I need Your help. I've asked for Your help so seldom about anything that ever mattered. So, I am asking You now. Please don't let me have cancer.

Amen.

Holding Pattern

The weekend came and went, leaving me to face Monday with a lump in my throat to match the one in my breast. Waiting to hear the results of the biopsy. *Maybe I will hear something today, or maybe it will be tomorrow. I need it to be today. I just need to know.*

As you wait, you hold on to everything you have. I held Kenny's hand a little tighter than usual, while holding my own breath. Everything around me was put on hold. Nothing was moving. Like a painting, everything was still and quiet. Even my

14

thoughts were motionless. Paralyzed in midair. As quickly as I allowed my mind to go there, I banished the thought. All thoughts. I was too afraid to be afraid. Too afraid to look in the mirror. Too afraid to rub my fingers on the area of my breast that was healing from the biopsy. I was sore, but the pain kept me in the present. *Right now, everything is fine. Until that phone rings, everything is fine. Until that phone rings, I don't have cancer.* I was unconvincing, even to myself.

Then the phone rang. It was the nurse calling to check on me. When I saw the number come up on my phone, I nearly jumped out of my skin. *Here we go.* But she told me right away that she wasn't calling with the results. She told me it would probably be Tuesday morning before I would hear from the radiologist.

So, I hung up the phone and stared out of the window in my office. Staring right back at me was the white brick wall of my neighbor's house. This would become a familiar scene for me in the months that followed. But in this moment, I felt relieved, if only temporary. *No cancer today.*

CHAPTER 2: THE DIAGNOSIS

A diagnosis is a very powerful thing, and it changes us forever.
But, we don't let it define us. We let it lift us.

The Call

I was in the bathroom first thing that Tuesday morning when my phone rang. I knew exactly who was calling. I saw the number flash on my iPhone screen, and that confirmed it. Straightaway, my heart began to race as my knees began to buckle. Panicked, I couldn't breathe.

"Hello."

"Hi Mrs. Sandlin. I'm the radiologist who performed the biopsy on you on Friday, and I would like to discuss the results, which we got back this morning. Is now a good time for you?"

"Um, yes. Please just tell me…do I have cancer?"

"The underlying result shows that it is positive for breast cancer."

Now that I knew for sure, I knew I didn't want to be alone.

"Could you give me five minutes? I need to get my husband in here so we can be on the call together?"

"Of course. I will call you back in five minutes."

Although Kenny was just downstairs, I called his cell phone. I knew it would be faster, and I needed faster. I told him it was cancer, and I heard myself say that sentence for the first time. It didn't sound right then, and still never does.

Moments after Kenny walked into our bedroom, the phone rang again. I climbed back on the bed, afraid my knees would give way. Then I put the call on speaker, hit the record button on my iPad, and simultaneously scrambled to take notes as my fingers shook around the pen.

"Hi! This is the radiologist again. Are you and your husband both on the call?"

"Yes. We are both here."

"So, the results of your biopsy show that you are positive for breast cancer. The type of cancer is invasive ductal carcinoma."

"What does that mean?"

"It means it started in the milk duct, which is a common type."

"OK. Keep going."

"Tumors are given a grade of 1-3 as to how aggressive they appear under the microscope, with 1 being the least aggressive and 3 being what appears to be an aggressive tumor that is multiplying quickly. Yours does have a grade of 3."

"Jesus!"

"Then we check to see what the tumor is sensitive to. Yours is what we call triple-negative, meaning that it is estrogen receptor-negative, progesterone receptor-negative, and HER2-negative."

"Is triple-negative a good thing or a bad thing?"

"It's neither good nor bad; it's just treated differently."

"So, it's treatable?"

"Yes."

"Sorry, I just have so many questions and I don't even know what I should be asking."

"That's perfectly normal. I know this is not what you wanted to hear, and I'm sure it's very overwhelming."

"That's putting it mildly."

It was all so technical and medical and foreign. There was no way to comprehend it all. The details about my diagnosis were just whizzing past my ears. I was only absorbing bits and pieces, so it was a good thing I was recording the call. Meanwhile, I kept watching Kenny's face. It had all of the emotions — all of them. Same as mine.

"So, what happens next? What do I need to do?"

"You will need to have a breast MRI so we can determine exactly how far the tumor extends in your breast, and to make sure all other areas in both breasts look fine. The MRI has already been ordered by your doctor and will be scheduled for later this week. You will also need to have an EKG. Then early next week, you will meet with a breast surgeon and an oncologist to discuss and coordinate your care and treatment plan. Also, genetic testing will likely be discussed, because a tumor with this profile is suggestive of a possible genetic etiology."

"OK. I'm on board. Whatever needs to happen, let's do it. The sooner, the better."

"Great. You will hear from the hospital shortly to schedule your MRI and EKG. You will also hear from the breast surgeon's office today to schedule an appointment with her."

When the call ended, Kenny and I just stared at each other. Neither of us were capable of forming words. I felt everything, yet nothing. It was like a blunt force trauma. There was blood, but no pain. As I breathed in, I could smell my own fear. It was pungent, like a mixture of blue cheese and grapefruit – two things I hate the most.

After sitting there on my bed for a few minutes, I realized I had three calls to make, and none of them would be easy. The first would be to Michael, then to my best friend Cheryl in California, and then to my daughter Kendall. That's when the tears started. Not mine, but theirs.

Michael

Starting with Michael, I could hear the cracking of his voice on the phone.

"Please. You have to promise me you're not going to do that. I don't want anyone to cry or be upset. This really sucks, but I just need everyone to stay positive. No tears. Nothing negative. Please. Promise me."

"OK. What do we need to do?"

"Nothing right now. I'm waiting to hear from the hospital and the breast surgeon's office. It sounds like things are going to move pretty fast. I need to call Cheryl and Kendall and let them know what's going on. Can I call you later?"

"Of course."

After our mom's death, Michael and I became closer than we had ever been. So, my diagnosis hit him very hard, especially given that we were still in the midst of our grief. We were in that together, and we would be in this together too. Kenny, Michael, and I dubbed ourselves the Three Musketeers. All for one and one for all. We did everything together. So, when I got cancer, we all got cancer.

Cheryl

Then I called Cheryl, my best friend forever. We have been friends since we were twelve years old, thanks to a random day when our moms ran into each other in the grocery store in Shreveport, Louisiana. That's where we lived. That's where I grew up.

I like to imagine our two moms (Marilynn and Marilyn) standing in front of the Pop-Tarts, having a brief chat, and sealing the deal. They decided they needed to get their girls together. It made sense. We went to the same school, played softball together, lived in the same neighborhood, and our houses were just a short bike ride away from each other.

A few days later, Cheryl called and invited me to her house to spend the night. And that was that. We have been best friends ever since.

Although she lives in California now, and I live in Texas, the miles have never kept us apart. We share an enduring bond of friendship that transcends the test of time and distance. We visit each other as often as possible, and we talk on the phone multiple times a week.

As I told her the news of my diagnosis, I could hear her breathe in slowly through her nose and then forcefully exhale through her mouth. It was a few seconds before she finally spoke.

"Wow! I can't believe it's cancer. I thought for sure you were going to call me and tell me that it wasn't. How do you feel?"

"I'm not even sure. My head is just spinning right now. There was so much to take in from my call with the radiologist. I don't even understand it all."

"Do you want me to come out there and…"

"No, no, no. Not just yet. As much as I'd love to see you, I've got to figure out all of these appointments, and I'm not sure about everything that's going to happen yet."

"So, what did they tell you? I mean, did they mention what stage the cancer is?"

"They think it's an early tumor. It started in the milk duct, which apparently is common. It's called invasive ductile carcinoma. The radiologist kept saying the tumor is very aggressive, so things are going to be moving fast. I know it sounds scary."

There it was again, that deep breath and exhale, holding back tears.

"Cheryl, please don't get upset. If you get upset, then I'm going to get upset, and I need to stay positive about everything. So, no tears. OK?"

"OK. I love you."

"I know. I love you too. Everything is going to be OK. I have to believe that."

"Yes, it will. Have you told Kendall yet?"

"No, I'm about to call her. I told her on Friday that it might be cancer, and I'm worried she's going to freak out."

"Hopefully, she will be OK. Call me later?"

"For sure."

Remember the movie, *Beaches*? Yeah, I didn't want that. (If you haven't seen the movie, I don't want to spoil it for you). Cheryl wanted to come visit me many times after my diagnosis, but each time I declined her offer. I was worried that if she came here, it would mean the situation was more dire than I could handle. I figured there would be plenty of time for visits — good ones — after I was on the other side of this. So, I wanted to save it until then.

Kendall

Then it was time to make the most difficult call of all. The one to my daughter Kendall. At first, I thought I might have to feed it to her in bite-sized morsels. I didn't think she could handle it all at once. I was wrong. She immediately pulled herself together and reminded me how strong she was.

"Hey woman! Have you heard anything yet?"

"Yes, and I am really sorry. I don't want to have to tell you this."

"What? Oh my God! Just tell me."

"The radiologist called this morning, and I am so sorry to have to tell you this, but I do have breast cancer."

"Oh no! I can't believe this is happening."

"It's OK. Please don't be upset. It's treatable, and I'm going to be fine. I have to be."

"Mommy, I love you so much. If anything ever happened to you…"

"No, no, no…don't go there. I love you too, and I will get through this. I promise. I am strong, and I am going to fight this with everything I have."

"You are the strongest person I know. And whatever you need, I will be there 100 percent. Whatever it is, you can count on me."

"I know I can, and that means everything to me. Please just try to stay positive. No tears. It's all I ask for now. I love you."

This daughter of mine. This woman. She amazes me every day. I wasn't going to let her be sad or scared for one minute, and she did the same for me. She was one of the people who needed me the most, and so I planned to stick around.

She continues to surprise me, and to show up for me, and to reinforce the fact that she is truly the strongest person I know. Much stronger than she realizes. In many ways, she stepped up and stepped into a role that had been vacated by my mom. Between Kenny and Michael, I was sandwiched in between a lot of testosterone. So, there were many times when I needed a different kind of comfort and tenderness. I needed Kendall's grit and determination around me. She made me brave. And she made me laugh — the kind that makes your belly hurt.

Joanne

There was one more call to make, but I just couldn't do it. I couldn't speak the words one more time that day. The more times the words left my lips, the more real they became. So, I asked Michael to make the call. It was to Joanne, our closest family friend.

I have always thought that people enter your life at the exact moment you need them to. From the day I lost my mom, Joanne has been in my life. She and my mom had been friends since the second grade. So, she was extremely distraught by the news of my mom's sudden and untimely death. Michael and I were in such pain and in need of comfort, and it was Joanne who swept in and wrapped her arms around us. We could feel this natural, immediate gravitational pull between us.

There is no doubt in my mind that my mom sent Joanne to us. And almost overnight, she became an integral part of our family.

I also consider Joanne my spiritual guide. And when you're going through cancer, a spiritual guide is a good thing to have. At the time, spiritual guidance was something I really lacked. Truth be told, I was still angry at God for taking my mom. But Joanne helped me find my way back. Faith by example. Her relationship with God is foremost in her life and completely unshakable. Her calming voice and the comforting tone of her words have a way of echoing in my heart.

Many times, she told me, *Sweetheart, put it in God's hands and leave it with Him. Remember, we are not in control. God is in control.*

I needed someone to make my problems feel a little lighter. A nurturing voice on the other end of the phone and in person. Someone to tell me everything was going to be OK. And Joanne believed it with all her heart. She believed in God. And she believed in me too. She wanted to lift my spirits, and often recited biblical verses. It was the purest expression of her emotions.

Nervous Energy

Nervous energy was starting to flow through my veins. My thoughts were coming in too fast with nowhere to go. They were just piling up like a traffic jam in my head. I knew I needed something to do. Take a shower. Have some coffee. Do something. Anything.

So, I transcribed my call with the radiologist. It always helps me to see things in writing. To see the actual words. It makes it easier to read and understand than to try and remember. Too much information and new terminology. Too much to absorb and deal with at the same time.

Journal: June 22, 2021

I have breast cancer. I've had to repeat those words several times today, and they still don't sound right. This was not supposed to happen. Today is my two-year Peloton anniversary and I'm in the shape of my life. But apparently, cancer don't care. The radiologist called me just as I woke up this morning. I recorded the call so I could transcribe it and put it in this big binder of information I am starting today. The most alarming word of the day, apart from "cancer," is the word "aggressive." The radiologist used it several times. I needed her to stop saying it. I needed her to stop saying all of it.

My world is about to turn upside down, and I am scared. This moment feels like the calm before an unprecedented storm. Batten down the hatches. Here we go.

As far as I knew, I didn't have any notable risk factors for cancer, or if I did, I thought they would have been extremely low. After all, I had a healthy lifestyle, and there wasn't much in terms of family history that mentioned cancer. So, how I got here made zero sense. But here I was anyway. Then there was the whole question about genetics. What did it all mean?

And what about the distinction between diagnosis and prognosis? That was difficult to reconcile. Not just at first, but during each phase of the journey, including the long road after. I am not even sure that it's possible to reconcile the two. The diagnosis is somewhat temporary, while the prognosis is ever-present.

. . .

As I went to bed that night — the night of my diagnosis — I began repeating the following words in my head: *I am more powerful than my diagnosis. I am more powerful than my diagnosis. I am more powerful than my diagnosis...*

Yes, a diagnosis is a very powerful thing, and it feels like it stops everything. Time itself has been suspended. And we know it will change us forever and in so many ways yet to be explained or discovered. But we must not let it define us. We need to let it lift us.

CHAPTER 3: SEARCHING FOR ANSWERS

I often search for answers in the lonely midnight sky...

Why?

The questions are only natural. You can't help it. You begin to doubt yourself and how you've been living your life, and the false sense of healthiness you thought you had mastered. And there it is. The most fundamental of all questions: *Why did this happen to me?* After everything I've already been through. The grief surrounding my mom's death. All the work I've done physically and emotionally. It seemed impossible that I was now facing a health crisis. A life-or-death crisis. *Cancer? Me?* It didn't even sound right. *I have cancer.* Those words didn't sound like my words. It didn't make sense. My mom didn't have cancer. Neither did my grandmothers. This can't be my story. It doesn't even fit.

You begin to question everything and look for an explanation. *What was my sin? What did I do wrong? What should I have done differently? What could I have changed or done better? How could I have prevented this?* No matter how much you question, the answer is always the same. You couldn't have stopped this because cancer don't care. It was in my genes. A predisposition. A ninja hiding in the darkness, dressed in black, waiting to strike. Waiting for its moment. Waiting to take me by surprise when I least expected it.

Repeatedly I asked myself (and God): *Why did this happen?* It just seemed so random, and a betrayal of everything I'd been doing to live a healthy life. To clear out the cobwebs and remove the deadly toxins. It's like my immune system had taken some unauthorized time off. It was AWOL. *Get back to work, you lazy bastard!*

I might always wonder why, but I couldn't focus on it. I had to keep everything in perspective. I couldn't allow myself to collapse into restless thoughts that didn't solve the problem at hand. The problem was cancer, and all my energy and resources were needed for the battle ahead. *Cancer be damned! You've met your match.*

Why Now?

The other part I continued to grapple with was the timing. It came on the coattails of losing my mom and the profound grief I had been living through for the past two years. I kept coming back to my healthy lifestyle and workout routine, and the irony of thinking I was the healthiest I had ever been, while instead, I was the most ill.

Like a broken record, the words just kept playing on repeat. I'm sure Kenny and Michael were tired of hearing them. *I eat healthy, work out like a maniac, don't drink, don't smoke, don't do drugs. I'm not overweight. I've done all the right things. Why cancer? Why now? Why me?*

Why Have I Been Chosen?

I guess it all comes down to this: *People plan, God laughs.*

So, why have I been chosen? This is something you ask yourself, and then you ask God. You remind yourself of the statistics. One in eight women will get breast cancer. I guess I drew the short straw. Maybe it's just as arbitrary as that. Like winning the lottery, only you don't get any money, and they might get to take your breasts.

Nonetheless, I'd like to believe that I was chosen for this for a reason. That's an attitude I adopted early on because how could *this* be for nothing? Everything happens for a reason, right? That's the simple explanation for life's most baffling circumstances. Perhaps the reason would be revealed in the journey itself.

Even in those early days, I knew I was going to share my experience. I had to. I thought it might make it a little less daunting for me, while giving others a peek behind the curtain of something so deeply traumatic that it might help them too.

While I will never know why cancer was put in my path, I was determined to give it a run for its money.

Cancer Don't Care

The very first thing I learned was that cancer don't care. And I realized there wasn't one thing I could have done differently to change what happened. Yes, it felt like a bad joke, and there were times when I thought, *who's in charge here? Let me speak to the manager. There must be a mistake.* Nope. This was not a mistake. God was in charge. And I would have to fight with every ounce of strength I had. I hadn't done anything wrong. I'd done everything right. But cancer don't care.

Cancer don't care about any of it. Cancer don't care who you are or what you've been through. Cancer don't care about your emotional state, or that you're grieving, or that you can't sleep at night, or that you have stress and anxiety, or that your whole world has already fallen apart. Cancer don't care about your workout routine or your diet. Cancer don't care about your lifestyle, your family, your finances, your creativity, your career, your goals. Cancer don't care about your business obligations, or that you have ideas and plans. Cancer don't care about your writing life and your ability to craft clever sentences or write poetry and prose. Cancer don't care that the timing is bad, or that you can't afford the disruption right now. Cancer don't care that you want to get organized, fix up your house, and move to Louisiana. Cancer don't care that you want to travel and climb mountains. Cancer don't care about your search for inner peace. Cancer don't care about your hair, or your skin, or how young you look. Cancer don't care who your parents are, or where you live, or where you went to college, or what kind of car you drive. Cancer don't care about your religion, or what your job is, or where you grew up. Cancer don't care how you dress, or how you look, or even if you have the right shoes. Cancer don't care what kind of shampoo you use, or your brand of toothpaste, or what

29

perfume you wear. Cancer don't care whether you're an introvert or extravert. Cancer don't care what your favorite movie is, or how you take your coffee. Cancer don't care about any of that. By all accounts, cancer is a narcissistic asshole.

It took me less time than you might think to arrive at this conclusion. There was no other justification or rationalization. It was beyond me. No matter how many ways I analyzed the situation, the answer was always the same. *CANCER DON'T CARE.*

Once you realize that, you can get past what happened and why it happened and start figuring out what you're going to do about it. Throwing your hands up in the air and calling it a day isn't an option. *Hell no!* You have to fight with everything you have. It's the classic battle between good and evil. You have to prove you're the stronger one. You have to evict this villain living inside you.

. . .

At first, I felt betrayed by my own body. *How could you do this to me after everything I've done for you? After everything I've given up for you?*

I felt betrayed and angry at God too. I felt that same anger when I lost my mom, but it was misplaced blame. It's anger that has no real place to go.

Betrayal is a sharp knife that cuts deeply. But this, this was a different kind of betrayal. One that was born within me. A betrayal of my body and health. *The call was coming from inside the house.*

Midnight Sky

In times of trouble or deep introspection, I often find myself looking out my bedroom window into the midnight sky. It's where I look for answers or some form of understanding. And in this moment, I had more questions than ever before. My life didn't feel like my life anymore. It had veered far off track, and I didn't know where I was going to end up.

Night after night, I stood at the window, peering through the plantation shutters at the midnight sky stretched out in front of me. My own slice of darkness.

Even as the house grew quiet, my head was still filled with noise. Deafening noise that swirled and swirled. I prayed, and I wished on little stars, obscured by the darkness. I reached out for my mom's outstretched hand, but it was too far away. I couldn't reach it. I couldn't reach her. The night was as vast as the ocean. Nothing but darkness as far as the eye could see.

I often imagine that what I see out that window is really the Pacific Ocean. I can feel the crisp salty air on my skin, and I can taste it on my lips. A lost paradise just beyond this terrifying forest. Palm trees waving in my direction. I wonder, *is this even my midnight sky, or am I standing in the middle of someone else's story?*

That's when I take a sharp turn towards God. Praying for strength. Praying for help. Praying to make it to the other side. Asking my mom to watch over me along with God. To stay with me a little while longer. To fight with me. To save me. To continue giving me life.

Preparing for the Fight

I think I had been secretly preparing for this fight. It was so secretive; I didn't even know what was happening. I was just doing it. Something was driving me to workout with the determination and obsessive style of an addict. I couldn't get enough. So, I don't think it just happened. Something inside just kept telling me to keep pushing myself harder.

Yes, on some level I had turned to working out as a way of coping with my grief, but it had become much more than that. Where did this drive come from? I believe it was heaven-sent. I like to imagine my mom and God conspiring and colluding on my behalf. Like a couple of personal trainers, they were encouraging me to challenge myself. To continue to make improvements and cheering me on with every accomplishment.

Just one more Peloton class. Just ten more reps. Just one more mile. You can do this. You are a fierce and stubborn warrior. Just keep moving, and you will be ready.

When I received my diagnosis, I felt like I was in the best possible condition for the fight ahead. I would even go as far as saying that I was in the best shape of my adult life. I was running for the first time in decades. With the wind at my back, I felt free and alive. It was meditative. It allowed me to clear my head of negative thoughts, process my emotions, and plan my future. To move my body with a vengeance, pushing through all of my anger, pain, and grief.

Little did I know I was being chased by cancer. No matter how fast I ran, it was outpacing me. With every step, it was getting closer and closer, and I was oblivious.

When it finally caught up with me, I had to lean a little harder on my inner strength, which would carry me through my diagnosis, treatment, recovery, and healing. This was a necessary, yet unconscious effort. It allowed me to slow down my thoughts just enough to be able to respond to everything that was coming at me. It was part of my punch-counterpunch strategy. And fortunately, it kicked in at the exact moment I needed it to.

So, where does inner strength come from? Some say it is part of who you are. Others say it comes from God. I like to believe it was both.

I've heard it said that inner strength also requires a healthy dose of courage. I can't say for sure where that comes from. All I know is you are forced to do difficult things that others will perceive as brave. It's what you do because you don't have a choice. You are under attack. So, you just summon the courage to face off against the very thing that threatens to take you down. Recognizing that courage and fear are two sides of the same coin.

Killer Boobs

I always thought I had nice boobs, but now I had *killer boobs*. They were literally trying to kill me. Just the idea of having to spend another day with a known murderer was more than I could take. *I don't want them anymore. Just take them.* I emotionally disconnected myself from them the moment I was diagnosed. I had to. They were no longer good; they were toxic. They were trained assassins, and they had to go.

Was it hard to disconnect like that? You'd think it would be, but it wasn't. Whenever I realize a situation is unchangeable, I manage to let it sink in and accept it. Don't get me wrong, it's not quite that easy. First, a brief panic ensues, accompanied by a lot of yelling and screaming, but once that's over, I move on.

The older I get, the more I understand the need for acceptance. In this situation, it was life-or-death acceptance. There was no other choice. If you have killer boobs, you just might have to preemptively kill those boobs instead. My sword was already drawn.

I'm not trying to minimize this at all. Just the thought of losing my boobs was extremely traumatic. I wasn't even sure what that meant or how it would look, or how I would feel, but I was willing to do whatever it took to fight this and stay alive.

Am I Going to Die?

The question at the core of this whole thing is the one we don't dare ask. The one we don't talk about. The real threat. *Am I going to die?* This is the question above all others. The gigantic elephant in every room. It follows you around the whole house and everywhere you go. And you do everything you can to ignore it, because acknowledging it makes it real. Makes it possible. And all you want is to make it go away. But there you are. Face to face with your own mortality. This overarching feeling of foreboding that you can't shake.

I learned not to dwell on it. My brain and my Kenny wouldn't let me. Anytime I brought it up, he immediately guided me away. It's not something anyone wants to talk about. So, most of the time, I locked those thoughts away. I didn't want to let them out to the universe. I was needed in this world, especially by Kenny,

33

Kendall, and Michael. I couldn't leave them. Not now and not like this. It wasn't my time, and I knew it.

I also knew that life isn't always on or off, in or out, up or down, alive or dead. But that's the way I prefer it, and that's what I so desperately wanted here. Confirmation that I would live. Confirmation that this wouldn't take me down. Still, no one around me could make any promises. *I have breast cancer.* Those were words I understood. But everything that came after had more ambiguity than my brain could manage. Unpredictability was laced into every moment, and every step brought more questions. *What's around the next corner? Where will this path take me? What's on the other side? Will I ever reach the other side?*

CHAPTER 4: GETTING ON WITH IT

You have to play the hand you've been dealt.
Folding is not an option.

Being a Researcher

For most of my adult life, I would consider myself an avid researcher. I enjoy the process of taking a deep dive into a subject and letting myself dig further and further down a rabbit hole. I love the organic nature of the meandering path, which often takes me places much farther away than I originally intended. It enables me to stumble upon the unexpected. To learn, explore, and gain knowledge, while fulfilling my innate curiosity. To take notes and look for the connective tissue.

But much to my surprise, I researched very little about this disease. *My* disease. *Don't Google stuff* was one of my new rules. I couldn't deal with statistics and outcomes and details about aggressive forms of cancer. It was too much. *Don't go there. Keep out!*

Later I would allow myself to Google some of the peripheral information, like *what to bring to chemo*, and *the side effects of chemo*, and *hair loss*, and *neuropathy prevention*, and *chemo brain*, and *managing nausea*, and a whole slew of other such topics. But for now, being in the dark about some of the more grueling details was where I needed to be. It was safer there. I could only deal with the things that were immediate. Everything else would have to wait.

Breast MRI

Three days after my diagnosis, I had an MRI of both breasts. This was my first official order, which was completed before I even met with my team of doctors. This was also my first MRI ever. I didn't know what to expect, except that I would be lying face down in a noisy machine for about forty-five minutes, with the strong likelihood I would feel claustrophobic.

My OBGYN prescribed a low dose of Diazepam to help me relax. I was nervous about taking it, so I broke it in half instead of taking the whole thing. I was having anxiety about taking anti-anxiety medication. Talk about ironic.

Kenny and Michael went with me. Michael was determined to be there for every appointment, except for those that only allowed one visitor because of COVID-19 restrictions.

When we arrived at the hospital, I was given some forms to fill out and asked to choose my music and aromatherapy options. I went with relaxing music and lavender mint, like it made any difference. I didn't think anything would help me relax, not even the Diazepam.

After changing into a hospital gown, I was given an IV so that my MRI could be administered with contrast and without. It's funny how you remember these small details, like the coldness of the MRI room, the warm blankets, and the friendly smiles on the technicians' faces. They looked like they didn't have a worry in the world, but I did. I had all the worries.

I was asked to lie face down with my arms stretched out in front of me like Superman, as the technicians positioned me onto the MRI machine. I kept my eyes closed the entire time. I had headphones on for the relaxing music and verbal commands. *Breathe in. Hold it. Relax.* I don't remember any of the relaxing music they promised, just the discomfort of my position, and the racing thoughts about what I was doing and why I was doing it. I don't think the Diazepam ever kicked in. It never stood a chance.

Afterwards, Michael suggested we have lunch. I wasn't hungry, but I knew I had to eat. We went to one of our favorite cafes. I wanted to sit outside, so that's what we did. Everyone wanted to do whatever I wanted to do. That's how you know when something is wrong. I ordered an Acai bowl with berries and coconut, and a hot green tea matcha latte with almond milk.

Michael insisted on chocolate chip cookies, so that happened too. I know it was delicious, but I couldn't even taste it. I was just ready to get home. My eyes were heavy. Perhaps the Diazepam had finally kicked in. I needed a nap. An escape nap.

Preparing to Meet the Team

It would be a dual appointment. I would see the breast surgeon first, then meet with the oncologist. The day before the appointment, I could feel this growing pit in my stomach. Emotionally, I was all over the place. Scared. Anxious. Nervous. You name it. I also realized it would soon be time to share this secret with a few more people, because I would need more help, support, love, encouragement, good vibes, happy thoughts, and a ton of prayers.

There was also the matter of my business clients and writing projects. I had several articles that were lingering out there, waiting for me to produce them. I wasn't sure how I could possibly deliver. Hard conversations were in my near future.

I was at a loss and in need of a brief diversion. Something to calm my nerves. So, I walked into my office, pulled out my copy of *A Poetry Handbook* by Mary Oliver, and read a few pages. Then a few more pages. Then I grabbed a notebook and a pen and wrote a poem loosely about mortality. *I guess there will be more of that. I guess there will be some darkness. I guess there will be lots of everything. I'm going to feel what I'm going to feel, and I will continue to spill my blood on page after page. That's just the way it is.*

> *I sometimes hear*
> *The strong sounds*
> *Of silent minds*
> *And the wistful feeling*
> *Of time slipping away*
> *As the solid roots*
> *And long leafy branches*

Devour all of God's creatures
As dusk gently gives way
To a new dawn

As I went to sleep that night, the call with the radiologist played over and over again in my head. The words she had used to describe my diagnosis were set on repeat, and I was still trying to digest them. It was impossible. So, I set my sights on tomorrow. There was a lot riding on tomorrow. I was anxious to meet my breast surgeon and my oncologist, two things I never thought I would need. I was anxious to learn more about my diagnosis. I was anxious to discuss the game plan. I was anxious to see their faces and read their expressions. And most of all, I was anxious to hear that I was going to be OK.

First Appointment

It was still the middle of COVID-19, when masks and social distancing were all the rage. Kenny and Michael sat down while I checked myself in. I was given the standard-issue clipboard with a stack of papers and forms to be filled out. As I turned to look for a seat, I was taken aback by my surroundings. There was yellow caution tape everywhere to partition off the seating for social distancing. It looked like a crime scene. It *was* a crime scene. *My* crime scene. This was the place where more forensic evidence would be gathered about me, my health, and my family history. We would discuss my diagnosis and prognosis, my treatment plan, and everything else about my case.

When I finished filling out the forms, I looked over at Kenny, who gave me a reassuring wink and a half smile. Then, trying not to stare, I glanced at the other women in the waiting room. There were only three, each with their own chosen head covering — a baseball cap, a scarf, and a turban. They all looked tiny, exhausted, and frail. As I sat there with my full head of hair, it hit me that soon I might be hairless, tiny, exhausted, and frail.

"Mrs. Sandlin? We're ready for you."

I stood up and headed in the direction of the nurse, as my entourage of two trailed behind me. We were led into the breast surgeon's office and seated at a small table. Kenny and Michael sat across from me. The nurse assured us that the doctor would be in shortly. Sitting there, taking in my surroundings and the gravity of what was about to go down, I could feel my heart beating faster.

"Are you OK?" asked Michael.

"No, not really. I can't believe where we are and why we're here."

"I know, but it's going to be OK," said Kenny.

"I hope you're right. I never in my wildest dreams expected to get cancer."

"Knock, knock," said the breast surgeon as she walked in and took the empty seat next to me.

As soon as she introduced herself, I could feel myself starting to sink. Even my vision became a little fuzzy. We were strangers, yet we were about to have one of the most difficult discussions of my life. I was scared to death, and I needed to know how we were going to eradicate this thing growing inside my breast.

There was a book on the table. It was called, *Be a Survivor, Your Guide to Breast Cancer Treatment,* by Vladimir Lange, M.D. Without skipping a beat, the doctor began flipping through the pages and pointing out specific sections.

As she flipped, I saw breasts and more breasts and other anatomical images and diagrams. She began to make a few select underlines and notes on some of the pages. She was talking, and I could hear her voice, but I understood very little of what she was saying. Not because of her, but because of me. The whole moment was surreal, and I was disconnected from the words. She might as well have been speaking Mandarin.

The more she spoke, the more I drifted further and further away. I didn't want to listen. Not to these words. They weren't *my* words. They must belong to someone else. I was nowhere near that table, or any table for that matter. I'm not sure where I was. I just knew I wasn't there. How could I be? Listening to those words that were not meant for me. They were someone else's words. Please return them to their rightful owner.

The only information I retained was that the tumor was 2.2-2.4 centimeters and that it was Stage IIB. Apart from that, I was told I needed to have an infusion port surgically placed near my left collar bone ASAP, chemo would begin right after that, and I was looking at either a lumpectomy, a mastectomy, or a double mastectomy. Oh yeah, and a genetic test would be ordered to determine whether I have a gene mutation.

I looked across the table at Kenny and Michael, wondering if they understood all of these words. Judging from the worried looks on their faces, yes, they understood the words, and that those words were now *my* words.

. . .

From there, we were escorted down the hall to the oncologist's office. Michael and Kenny stepped out while I changed into the obligatory examination gown and answered some questions with the nurse. I recognized her accent immediately.

"You're from New Orleans, aren't you?"

"Yes, how did you know?"

"I'm from Louisiana, and I know a New Orleans accent when I hear one."

"Born and raised, girl. I was born and raised in New Orleans."

"I'm going to take this as a good sign."

Just then, Kenny came back into the room to wait with me. We sat there, both of us unable to speak. Then there was a knock on the door.

"Come in."

It was the oncologist. She bounced into the room with an air of optimism and positivity that I found instantly encouraging.

After a brief introduction, she looked deeply into my eyes and said, "You are going to be OK."

There was something about the way she looked at me and her matter-of-fact tone that made me believe her. *I was going to be OK.*

Then she drew a diagram and wrote a few words on a piece of

paper, all of which confirmed what we already knew. *Breast cancer. Invasive ductal carcinoma. Triple-negative. Stage IIB.*

The treatment plan would be chemo for the next six months, followed by surgery. It would start with twelve rounds of chemo given once a week for twelve consecutive weeks. During that time, I would be getting infusions of Taxol and Carboplatin. Then I would have a few weeks off, followed by four rounds of Adriamycin and Cytoxan, which would be given three weeks apart.

That was the first time I realized that not all chemo was the same. I had no idea there were different kinds. I just thought chemo was chemo. I had never heard the words Taxol, Carboplatin, Adriamycin, or Cytoxan before in my life. So, they meant nothing to me. All I knew was that this treatment strategy was meant to aggressively shrink the tumor that was aggressively growing inside me.

Scary Words

It seemed like there was no end to the scary words. And they just kept throwing them out there for me to catch. They weren't part of my vernacular, but somehow, I tried to work them in. And I did so without overthinking them. I tried to use them in sentences with the same ease at which they were flung at me. I learned to repeat them. To ingrain them in my everyday life. I sat with them. I stared at them. I hated them. And I accepted them, because I didn't have a choice.

Here are just a few of them: *breast cancer, tumor, invasive ductal carcinoma, aggressive, fast replicating, triple-negative, Stage IIB, gene mutation, infusion port, chemo, surgery, lumpectomy, mastectomy, double mastectomy.* Oh yeah, and let's not forget *hair loss* and *bald.*

I still have trouble with some of the medical terminology and what it all means. Even as I write this, I'm looking up terms like *risk of recurrence* and *life expectancy.* I don't think I will ever stop researching these terms, even though I established a *do not Google* rule for myself early on. It's still a lot to wrap my head around.

And none of it sits right with me.

Positives & Negatives

Everything gets broken down quickly into binary code. You are positive for this and negative for that. It sounds so simple, but each plus and minus brings a new set of issues. And positive isn't necessarily a good thing. Sometimes it is just affirming, which runs counter to the ideas we have about positives and negatives. So, you constantly ask what positive means in this context and that. Positive for breast cancer. Triple-negative breast cancer.

Positivity. This I understood. I had to stay positive, which meant stripping away all the emotional negativity. Negative thoughts. Negative people. I didn't need them or want them around me in any capacity. So, I cleaned house. I refused to allow negative thoughts and fears to creep in and cause the inevitable downward spiral. The point of no return. I knew I had to shoot down those thoughts the moment they entered my air space. They served no purpose, and I couldn't risk the drain of valuable resources.

But there were moments, and days when it seemed impossible. Those thoughts would bubble up and take over. Streaming and screaming feelings that said, *something very bad has happened, and something even worse might be lurking around the next corner.* So, whenever I realized that I was racing down that road, I stopped myself in my tracks.

That's why I established the *no tears allowed policy* within my close inner circle from day one. If I wasn't crying, they couldn't be crying. It wasn't the time for tears. It was time for positivity, and I wanted to surround myself with as much of it as humanly possible. If, God forbid, the time came when we needed tears, then we would reevaluate. But for now, and until further notice, no tears were allowed.

CHAPTER 5: THE CALM BEFORE THE SHIT STORM

Thinking positive means you sometimes have to wear sunglasses in the rain.

Letting It Sink In

Right after my diagnosis, things started moving pretty fast. There was no time to catch my breath. No time to think. I had tasks to complete, phone calls to make, appointments to set, and chores to be done. There were many fast-paced steps, and they all required my attention. I kept telling myself that it was only a task list, and I could handle it. *Remember, you're a taskmaster. Just keep checking boxes and working the list. Don't think. Thinking is dangerous.*

Because of the urgency of the situation, there wasn't much time to let my diagnosis sink in. Forget processing the words or conducting research. You only get a few minutes to hear the words, absorb them, accept them as true, and just get on with it. That can be a good thing though. No time for self-pity. You just get moving. Treatment comes at you very fast, and you have to be ready to go.

Meanwhile, emotions run rampant through your body. You feel all of them. Terrified, overwhelmed, shocked, stunned, anxious, nervous, numb. *This can't be real. This can't be happening. Not to me. I must be dreaming.* You pinch yourself only to find that you are wide awake. You find yourself in some alternate reality. *How did I get here, and when do I get to go back home? This isn't where I am supposed to be.*

Then there are the emotions of those around you. Somehow you are responsible for those too. Suddenly you find yourself at the center of some new solar system, and everyone in your orbit is trying to figure out what they should to be doing. Looking for clues of what you might need and how to help you. I was acutely aware of the unspoken, shared worry of Kenny, Kendall, and Michael. I could see it on their faces and hear it in their voices. They tried to hide it, but they were terrible at hiding. It became my job to keep reassuring them that I was OK. And that I was going to make it through, no matter how tough things might get.

They knew me, and they knew my determination. So, when this thing *happened to me*, which is how I saw it, it all became about making it to the other side. And getting to the other side meant I had to pool all my resources. It was going to take grit, persistence, positivity, strength, perseverance, tenacity, prayer, hope, and a whole lot of love. And I was prepared to do whatever it took. The contract was drawn up and signed in blood. *My blood.*

Positivity

I have always believed that thinking positive means you sometimes have to wear sunglasses in the rain. It's a simple way of describing this complex ordeal, and that's because attitude is so important. Positivity is a choice. So is negativity. And there was no way I was going to feel sorry for myself. Not for one second. There wasn't time for that, and it wasn't my style. Admittedly, positivity hasn't always been my go-to move either, but something told me it was the only way to go in this situation, and so I listened. Negativity would have only further poisoned the well, and what I needed to do was to obliterate the poison, not give it a reason to grow.

I can't overemphasize the power of positivity and the way it makes you feel. From the beginning, it was the image I wanted to portray, even on my worst days. Yes, my fear was often on full display, but it was equally laced with positivity. I did this for the people around me, but I also did it for myself. I needed to believe my own bullshit, drink my own Kool-Aid, fake it until I made it.

By approaching each challenge with positivity, I was subsequently reducing my feelings of negativity. It was a simple formula, and it worked. Don't get me wrong, I had my moments and my days when no matter how hard I tried, I just couldn't tap into that positivity. But damn if I didn't try.

Putting My Affairs in Order

Before things got any crazier than they already were, I thought I'd better call my attorney and put my affairs in order. It seemed like a practical next step after receiving a cancer diagnosis. It gave me a time-sensitive project. A welcome diversion. A way for me to call the shots and make some decisions.

So, I placed a call to my attorney the day after my diagnosis and asked him to draft the appropriate documents. He understood the urgency and was able to move at my pace, which was like lightning. He was even kind enough to let me, Kenny, and Michael come to his house and sign the documents on a Saturday.

It was a beautiful June day, the kind that feels like vacation weather. The attorney's family was swimming outside and having a good time, while I was inside signing my last will and testament, medical directives, and powers of attorney. The dichotomy of the moment was almost laughable.

I wanted to be outside, laughing and enjoying myself too. Instead, I was staring at words on pages with red flags showing me where to initial and where to sign. Life was continuing to go on all around me and without me. I was taking a forced leave of absence, and making my wishes known.

. . .

Later that day, I told Kenny we needed to get the house organized. That I wanted to put my affairs in order at home too.

"You're putting too much pressure on yourself," said Kenny.

"I just feel like we should take this time to get some things done. You know, before the storm."

"You have a lot on your plate already, and I don't want you stressed out. Remember, it's not good for you. Just relax, and we will figure everything out together as we go."

"I would just feel better if I knew the house was in order."

"There's nothing else to get in order. The house is fine, and you are going to be fine. You're not going anywhere. So, just relax and let it go."

The Binder

One of the things the radiologist suggested to me at the end of the diagnosis phone call, was to put a binder together. She told me there was going to be a lot of information that I would want to keep together and organized. Boy, she wasn't kidding. There were medical records, pathology reports, doctors' notes, imaging orders, medication information, insurance correspondence, receipts, nutritional information, helpful resources…and the list goes on and on.

This was a project I could lose myself in, and frankly, I needed to get lost. It started with the search for the perfect 3-ring binder on Amazon. You would think that would be easy, and for most people it would be, but not for me. After a long search, I found one I liked and placed the order. But when it arrived, I didn't like it. So, I ordered another one. Didn't like that one either. So, I ordered a third one. The first one was too small, and the second one was too flimsy, but the third one was just right. *Just like Goldie Locks and the Three Bears.*

Then there were the dividers, sheet protectors, and Sharpie markers. Not just any Sharpies. They were my mom's Sharpies, pulled directly from the decorative cup that sat on her desk and now resides on mine.

I just needed to stay busy. Organize the growing stack of paper in my office. Relish in my creation of the perfect binder. Keep it up to date. File every document and piece of paper. Put everything in the right place. Share it with Kenny so he will know where to find something if he needs it.

I was so proud of that binder. It was supposed to organize the chaos, but instead, I somehow managed to make chaos out of order. Everything was all neat and orderly until a few weeks later when my chemo brain started to misfire. After that, I can't say exactly what happened. Pieces of paper were stuck in random sections of the binder. I tried to create some new sections when needed, and that was mostly a mess too. *Oh well. I tried.*

The Wig

My oncologist told me I would start to lose my hair soon after my first round or two of chemo. I was no stranger to the concept. I understood the basic correlation between going through chemo and hair loss. I had seen this on TV shows and in movies, just not up close and personal. And certainly not from my own reflection in the mirror. Still, hearing that I would be losing my hair — sooner rather than later — was news that landed with a thud. No need to process; this is how it was going to be.

You'd think I'd be way more upset about losing my hair, but oddly that bothered me very little. Besides, there were too many big-ticket items to focus on. After all, it was only hair.

So, rather than dwelling on the inevitable, I scheduled a wig consultation. It was the sensible thing to do. And although there were many choices out there — free or paid, synthetic or human, this color or that — I knew what I wanted. I wanted human hair that looked as much like my own hairstyle and color as possible. I didn't want anyone to be able to tell it was a wig, or that I didn't have a full head of hair, or that anything had changed. And for that, I was willing to pay a price. *Sky's the limit.* Besides, since I would no longer need to have my hair colored and cut every six weeks, I figured this wig expense would be a wash. I was treating myself. I was controlling this. I deserved this.

Journals

I have journaled for most of my life, so journaling about my cancer journey came naturally. I wanted to document everything as best as I could. I wanted to be able to look back and remember

— the good, the bad, the bald. I wanted to get it all down, just in case. Things were happening fast, and the ground beneath me had already started to shift. I wanted to capture all of it on paper as fast as I could. Later, chemo brain would take over, and my writing might be more like scrambled eggs. So, I reached for my journal and started to write it all down. Not just the day-to-day happenings, but the emotional impact everything was having on me and those around me.

My goal was to write something every day. That never worked out. Some days were too busy. Other days, I didn't feel like it. And other days I was too riddled with fatigue and nausea to even sit up in the bed, much less hold a pen and let my thoughts flow out onto the page. Nonetheless, I managed to get something out of myself at least once a week, and that was enough.

During the early days following my diagnosis, I also started keeping a separate health journal for logging appointments, writing down discussions with my doctors, keeping track of reactions and side effects to chemo and other medications, and all other related events. I knew I wouldn't be able to remember everything later, and I might need to refer to it from time to time.

The physical act of writing it all out on paper was critical for me. I thought I could later compare the health log with the emotional side of things. Compare and reflect on what was happening physically to my body along with the emotional side effects. And that's exactly what I have done in writing this book.

Overwhelmed

It doesn't take much to feel completely overwhelmed. You've been handed a diagnosis, along with a laundry list of new vocabulary words and terms. You are meant to internalize them. Instantly your everyday speech starts to change. Sensory overload. Do this. Write down that. Call this number. Make this appointment. Buy this. Stay away from that. *Aggressive. Invasive ductal carcinoma. Stage IIB. Triple-negative. Chemotherapy. Lumpectomy. Mastectomy. Double mastectomy. Risk factors. Genetic testing. Survival rate.*

It was hard to grasp how different my life had become in such a short time. I tried to keep it somewhat normal by working and staying productive, but I couldn't focus. Work seemed frivolous. And I still hadn't shared the news with anyone outside of my inner circle. I wanted to keep this private a little while longer.

So, I filled in the gaps with the only things I could do. The only things that were in my control. I rode my Peloton. Not like my previous Peloton rides, but Peloton rides with a vengeance. Angry peddle strokes with a cadence as fast as I could push myself.

I also spent time on some creative endeavors. I wrote a poem or two. Played my drums. Bought some art. Yes, I bought some art. Having cancer inspires you to do things you've never done before.

One day, not long after my diagnosis, I commissioned a piece of art by an extremely talented friend of mine. We had known each other since our freshman year at LSU. During the pandemic, she began sharing her art on social media. Something about it just spoke to me. And she spoke to me, with that familiar southern drawl that beckoned me home. I can't explain it. I just needed to own a piece of it, so I reached out and she obliged.

Then, a few months later, I bought another piece of art. This one was by a distant cousin of mine. A cousin I had never met. But as cousins, we connected with each other through social media. And her art spoke to me too, so I wanted to have one of her pieces around me.

Admittedly, neither piece of art has been given its rightful place on the walls of my house, but they will. At the time, I just leaned them against a wall in our guest room, as if they were somehow temporary. Everything felt temporary. Nonetheless, these purchases represented a sense of control. My ability to make some decisions. To trust my impulses.

It was true, I had entered a new space where I had very little control. Kenny was trying hard not to treat me any differently. He wanted to keep things as normal as possible. But I finally had to tell him that this was anything but normal. Everything had changed, and so I needed him to change a little too. To be a bit nicer to me. Not that he wasn't being nice, but just that I needed something extra now. You would think after thirty-five years, he would pick this stuff up on his own, but I still had to tell him. And that's OK.

I was afraid I might lose myself, so I needed him to keep things steady. I didn't know where I was, much less what was going on. *We're not in Kansas anymore,* I thought out loud. Only it wasn't my voice I heard. It was my mom's.

Eat the Damn Cookie

I thought I should try doing something *normal,* so I accepted an invitation to a business meeting. It seems completely ridiculous as I look back, but at the time, I knew it would be my last one for a while, so I went anyway. I might as well have been in outer space because I sure as hell wasn't present at that meeting. I had to sit there and smile and be engaging and pretend that everything was OK. *It most certainly was not OK.* But somehow, I got through it.

When it was over, I said a quick goodbye, made a mad dash to the parking lot, and jumped in my car.

On the way home, I felt the rush of everything that was happening. It was all moving so fast that I needed a moment to stop, slow down, and catch my breath.

I realized I was close to one of my favorite cafes. So, I pulled into the parking lot, exited my car, went inside, and grabbed a table. I knew I had to sit there and relax for a minute. Then I glanced over and saw one of their addictive chocolate chip cookies looking back at me. So, I ordered one, along with my standard hot green tea matcha latte with almond milk.

When the server set my order down in front of me, I knew it was much more than a little nosh. This was about stopping the manic trajectory of my racing thoughts and taking a moment just for me. A moment to slow down, pause, and breathe.

As I took that first bite of the cookie, I felt the stress start to melt away, just like the chocolate on my tongue. It was an important reminder not to turn off that inner voice when your body tells you that you need a moment. You have to listen to it. Stop the car and stop the madness. You don't have to keep moving in lockstep with your anxiety. Break away and break free. No regrets. Eat the damn cookie.

CHAPTER 6: GEAUX TIME

Seeing the path before you is not enough.
Pack your bag!

Warp Speed

It's strange how quickly things went from the slow pace of me trying to talk myself out of having a lump just a few weeks earlier, to everything moving at warp speed. It had taken some ingenuity to push my way to the front of the line when it mattered most. I was already in fight mode and doing that thing I do so well — making things happen. I was speeding through the middle of chaos without hitting the brakes. Running headfirst into the great unknown. I traded in my laces for slip-on shoes. When you need to move fast, you can't afford to stop and lace up your shoes. You have to wear slip-ons. Mine were Vans.

Even as fast as everything was moving, there was also a lot of waiting in between. Waiting to schedule my MRI and echocardiogram. Waiting to meet the breast surgeon and oncologist. Waiting to clear health insurance hurdles. And I've never been very good at waiting. I'm impatient by nature, so waiting made me anxious. Every minute I spent waiting, reinforced my lack of control. I could feel it slipping away. I was relinquishing the steering wheel and becoming the passenger in my own car.

Diagnosis to Chemo

There were only three short, jam-packed weeks between my diagnosis and my first round of chemo. There were lots of hurdles to clear and tasks to be checked off my ever-growing list.

It looked like this:

June 22:   *Diagnosis*

June 25:   *MRI of breasts*

June 28:   *First appointment with my breast surgeon
and oncologist*

June 29:   *Baseline lab work and wig consultation*

July 2:   *Port placement procedure*

July 6:   *MRI of liver and echocardiogram*

July 13:   *Chemo round 1*

Oh, and I also managed to attend a business networking event a few days after I was diagnosed. That night was ridiculous. I thought it would be the most ordinary thing I could do. *Nope.* I was, at best, a fish out of water. The words *I have cancer* were on the tip of my tongue, but I didn't tell anyone. I didn't even really talk to anyone except for this one friend. I picked her because she is quiet like me, and I needed quiet. I opened my mouth a couple of times, thinking I might be able to tell her, but it was no use. I couldn't even sound out the words. It was time to go. *Was I even there? Maybe it was a dream.*

Going Public

Do you go public with a private moment? In my case, the answer was a resounding *yes.* I knew this almost as soon as I was diagnosed. I figured, if there was the slightest chance that someone was listening and could benefit from my experience, that it was important for me to share my journey. Besides, it would have been unlike me to suddenly go silent on social media.

Over the previous two years, I had shared my grief. Then I shared my fitness journey, while encouraging others to keep moving and make healthy choices too. Then the pandemic hit, and I shared videos of myself as I walked through my neighborhood. I shared my views about life, health, working out, grief, being alone, priorities, anxiety, stress, self-care, you name it. And then, almost poetically, those messages naturally dovetailed into my new message without skipping a beat.

So, it made sense to make a video announcement. Raw and unedited. I was only twelve days away from my first chemo infusion, and I wanted to do it before losing that first strand of hair.

Sitting alone in my office, with my iPhone in my left hand, I pointed it in my direction and hit the red record button. *Here goes nothing.*

> *This is something I never thought in my wildest dreams I would be making a video about, but here we are. First, there are things we self-diagnose ourselves with, and I've done that my whole life. I'm OCD, ADD, and maybe a little dyslexic. I have high-functioning anxiety and high-functioning depression — all manageable stuff. But the thing that kicks us in the ass, is a medical diagnosis. I will cut to the chase here; I have just been diagnosed with breast cancer. And wow! I didn't see that one coming. I feel like I'm in the prime of my life. I exercise six days a week, I eat very clean, I don't drink alcohol, I don't do drugs, I don't smoke. I live a very healthy life, but cancer don't care. Cancer don't care…*

I promised to share my journey and post updates about what's going on and how I'm doing. I also encouraged people to be diligent when it comes to anything that might seem abnormal for their own bodies. And to not ignore the warning signs. *If something doesn't feel right or you don't feel right, go to the doctor!*

I played back the video to make sure there weren't any technical glitches. All looked good. Then I took a deep breath, opened my Facebook app, and posted the video with this preamble: *Life is full of unexpected, unscripted moments that you never thought would happen to you, but here we are.*

Oh, the irony of putting out all those videos promoting health and fitness, and now here I was announcing my breast cancer diagnosis.

Immediately the comments and messages started pouring in. Then my phone started blowing up with texts and calls. *I had put it out there, and now there's no going back.*

I knew I had done the right thing by posting the video. My mom would have disagreed. She wouldn't have understood my need to go public with something so personal and private. *Why would you put something so personal like that on Facebook? Some things are meant to stay private.* She wouldn't have understood it until probably months later. She would need time to get used to it — used to me having cancer — and then one day, she'd tell me that she understood why I shared it. She might even say, *I'm proud of you for opening yourself up like that.*

This was my story, and I wanted to tell it on my terms. Authentic and unedited. You can see the terror written all over my face. My vulnerability on full display. But my message was clear. It was one of hope, positivity, and powering through no matter how rough things might get.

As my Maw-Maw Pearl would say, *never let the bastards get you down.* In spite of the diagnosis, I wasn't about to let it get me down. I wanted to show people that I was OK. Petrified, but OK.

Questions Everyone Asks

Inquiring minds want to know, and I had no problem telling. Anything I was asked, I answered. People would often preface their questions by saying, *if it's too personal, you don't have to answer.* But I didn't mind at all. I was an open book.

Most questions came from women, although I did receive a few from men. I think men were a bit hesitant to ask me about my breasts without feeling weird about it. Maybe I'm wrong.

The most common questions were: *Did you find a lump? How big was your tumor when you were diagnosed? What stage is your cancer? Does cancer run in your family? What kind of breast cancer do you have? Will you be having surgery? What kind of surgery? Will you have chemo?*

Will you have radiation?

At first, whenever I retold my story, I did so with a *stick-to-the-facts* kind of style, omitting much of the emotion and fear unless I was specifically asked about it. Just skimming the surface. It was easier that way. Just the facts. It kept me somewhat removed from what was actually happening. Almost like it was happening to someone else. An armor of words to shield me from danger. By sticking to the facts, it helped me feel like I was controlling my own narrative. I had it down and could easily recite it by heart.

Say No to Pink

As soon as I went public, I could feel the pink rolling in. It was everywhere. People commented on my Facebook posts with pink hearts, sent me text messages with pink emojis, and sent me various pink gifts. I know they meant well, but I just couldn't do it — embrace the pink and the solidarity of this official breast cancer color. It wasn't for me. It still isn't. I didn't need or want the pink ribbons either.

So, I had to stop the flow of pink. And there was no easy way around it. I had to be blunt. And that's OK, because people understood. *Just so you know, I'm not doing the pink ribbon thing. Besides, I never wear pink because it makes me look like a giant bottle of Pepto-Bismol.*

I realize that not everyone shares my thoughts on pink, but I had to be true to myself. This was something small that I could control, and saying *no* was a powerful thing. I knew that soon I would be losing my hair, and soon I would look like a walking billboard for breast cancer. I didn't need the addition of pink ribbons as proof.

Port Placement Surgery

We arrived at the hospital at 6:00 in the morning. Kenny and Michael were both with me. The rest is pretty much a blur, except for this. I was lying in the hospital bed, waiting for the breast surgeon to come in and talk to me before this minor surgery. When she walked in, she positioned herself at the foot of my bed and began rubbing my feet. An instinctive impulse. That's what my mom did for me when I was in labor with Kendall. And that's what I did for Kendall when she was in labor with my first two grandsons, Jake and Robbie. Then in 2019, the tables turned completely around. It was me gently rubbing my mom's feet as she laid there motionless in her hospital bed.

I closed my eyes as the doctor continued to rub my feet, imagining my mom's long fingers around my toes. Imagining my mom's voice telling me everything was going to be OK. Imagining her telling me I would be OK. That's the last thing I remember before going under.

. . .

On the drive home from the hospital, I started feeling sleepy and nauseous from the anesthesia. As soon as we got home, I climbed into bed and slept on and off for the rest of the day and night. I was a sore and had no appetite. The next day was the same. But by the following day, I was much better. I was also stir-crazy and needed to get out of the house. So, Michael took me to Whole Foods to pick up a few things. He needed to feel useful, and I needed to let him.

Having my port put in was the last step before chemo. Things were starting to get very real, and the next step would be a dubious one.

False Sense of Euphoria

I often break up my weeks into winners and losers. The winner for me the week between getting my port put in and starting chemo, was that the procedure caused very little discomfort. The loser was my false sense of euphoria. I'd been trying to maintain this level of positivity, and I'd done a decent job so far. But now

I was starting to get a little scared, nervous, and anxious. I didn't know what it was going to be like to have that first chemo infusion, or what effect it would have on me. It was fear of the unknown on steroids. Trying to stay upbeat was exhausting. I was struggling to maintain this higher altitude. I thought the air was meant to be thinner up here, but it felt as thick as mud.

Pre-Chemo Anxiety

How do you prepare yourself for that first round of chemo? I had no idea. The night before my first round, I was so anxiety ridden that I couldn't sleep. Instead, I busied myself in my office trying to figure out what to bring with me to the Infusion Center the next morning. I came up with a whole list of items and painstakingly packed them into three separate bags that I will forever refer to as my *giant bags of crap*. The bags contained a blanket, a pillow, a jacket, extra socks, a baseball cap, ice gloves and ice socks (to help with neuropathy), a water bottle, snacks, a book, a notebook, a pocket planner, an iPad, an iPhone charger, and earbuds.

When it came down to it, the only things I needed were the ice socks and ice gloves. Still, my need to pack was driven by my anxiety. It gave me something else to focus on instead of what was waiting for me the following morning. That's when poison would be entering my body and having its way with my cells. Rooting out the evil lurking within my breast.

I hoped I would wake up the next morning and Kenny would tell me it was all a dream. All of it. The part where my mom died. The part where I had breast cancer. But, as the clock ticked on, the more real it all became.

I was scared, but there were so many other emotions pouring out of me at the same time. I felt so much, yet nothing at all. There was this enormous feeling of dread mixed with urgency. *Let's go. Wait, not yet.*

I knew the moment I sat in the chemo chair, that I would be leaving the old me behind. Poison would be dripping its way into my veins and running rampant throughout my body. Another life-altering scenario playing itself out right before my eyes. *How can so much happen to one person to completely rip their world apart — not once, but twice — in a little over two years?*

I thought it might help to make a short video and share what I was feeling on the eve of my first chemo. It went something like this.

> *I'm still trying to comprehend everything, even though none of it feels remotely connected to me. Tomorrow, I will start chemo, and I have no idea what kind of effect that will have on me. I'm having a lot of fear about all the side effects, and whether they will happen to me, and how soon they will happen. I don't want to feel sick, and I don't want to look sick. At the same time, I have to stay positive even though I'm having all of this fear, and that causes a lot of anxiety.*

I was so terrified as I spoke the word. *Chemo.* It still didn't feel like one of my words. As soon as it left my lips, I could see it hanging there in midair, taking its time before landing.

Pre-chemo anxiety is something I would feel during the days leading up to each infusion. It hit me especially hard the day and night before. I would try to mentally prepare for the surrender by forcing various distractions, like sitting in my office, looking through books, and writing in my journal. Trying to encourage the creative flow of something beautiful.

But the night before my first round was the most difficult. No matter how much I read to better inform myself about what to expect, the less I understood. I knew that poison was going to be injected into my body to kill the poison that was already in my body. It sounded barbaric. And I knew my hair was going to start falling out. And I knew I was going to feel like crap. And I knew that prayers indeed were needed.

Pre-Chemo Ride

I began each chemo day by riding my Peloton. It is a ritual I started on the morning of my first round of chemo and continued until the morning of my final round. It was nonnegotiable. A firm commitment to myself. Besides, my oncologist said working out was a very good thing, so that's all I needed to hear. I had also read that working out before each infusion helps prepare the veins for chemo. It allowed me to do something healthy on the same day I was allowing dangerous poison to wreak havoc on my body. Toxins in. Toxins out. So, that was the routine I followed religiously.

Still, I didn't know how chemo would affect me in terms of my workouts, so I had to play it by ear. At first, I stuck to my regular forty-five-minute ride routine, followed by a five-minute post-ride stretch. But as the weeks went on, the length of my rides diminished with each round of chemo. By the morning of my final round, I was only able to ride for ten minutes. Picture a sloth on a Peloton. That was me. Slowly pedaling. All my energy zapped away.

First Chemo

It doesn't matter how much you read, or what they tell you; nothing prepares you for that first round of chemo. The psychological aspects alone are enough to scare the shit out of you. *Will I feel it? Will I feel the poison entering my body? Will I feel like I've been poisoned?*

I was told I could have two visitors with me at the Infusion Center. So, with Kenny and Michael in tow, I drove us to the hospital.

We walked in with my three giant bags of crap. Someone should really call you before your first round of chemo to set your expectations and tell you what you need bring. We must have looked ridiculous.

Upon reaching the Infusion Center, we were told that Kenny

and Michael had to tag team, as I could only have one visitor with me at a time. Kenny told Michael to go with me first so he could grab some coffee. I must have won the lottery that day, because I was given a brand-new private room, complete with a big comfy recliner that was heated and vibrated. *Woohoo!*

Moments later, my infusion nurse waked in and told me everything that was going to happen.

"First, we are going to access your port and flush it with saline, which you will probably taste. Then we're going to draw a little blood and send it to the lab. If the bloodwork looks good, then we will order your chemo."

"OK. How long does it normally take to get the OK from the lab?"

"Not too long today. Probably about thirty minutes or so. As soon as we get that back and order your chemo, we can start you on your pre-chemo meds."

"Oh, what kind of pre-chemo meds will I be getting?"

"We'll give you some Benadryl, Prevacid, Zofran, and a steroid — all through your port. Then we will give you the Taxol followed by the Carboplatin. Once that's complete, we will flush your port with saline again, then you can go home."

"So, everything will take a few hours?"

"I would say it's about four hours or so from the time you arrived until the time you leave. Would you like to order lunch? I can bring you a menu."

It all sounded so run-of-the-mill. Just a regular day in the Infusion Center. Chemo and lunch. Nothing to see here. Everything was fine and normal. Only nothing was fine or normal.

. . .

It was go time. My port was accessed and flushed with saline. Instantly, the salty taste made me want to gag. Later I would learn to pop a curiously strong Altoid peppermint into my mouth just before the saline was plunged into my port.

In a flash, my blood was drawn and sent to the lab, and the

nurse reappeared to let me know that all looked good, and my chemo had been ordered.

Then it was time for my premeds. Within seconds of receiving the Benadryl through my port, it hit me, and my speech began to slur, and I felt all kinds of woozy. The immediate relaxation washed over me.

Then Michael tapped out. It was Kenny's turn to be my plus-one.

"Hey there! Where have you been all my life? Come on in."

"Did they give you something? You seem a little out of it," Kenny said.

"Yes, it's the Benadryl. Not just any Benadryl. Heavy-duty Benadryl. They gave me some other pre-chemo drugs too, but I can't remember what they are."

Within minutes of Kenny walking in, it was chemo time. The infusion nurse walked back into the room, this time wearing the equivalent of a hazmat suit.

"Wow, that looks pretty serious," I said.

"Yes, I know, but it's standard protocol when administering chemo."

Kenny helped me put on my ice socks and ice gloves. Then I braced myself.

"We are going to start the chemo now," the nurse said. "Are you ready?"

"As ready as I will ever be. Let's do it."

I was so cold from the socks and gloves. I felt like ice-cold water was moving through my veins along with the poison. I was so sleepy from the Benadryl. I could feel myself starting to doze off. My head was bobbing, and my eyes were heavy. I knew it was common to sleep during chemo, but I was too tense, even with the Benadryl.

When my lunch arrived, Kenny helped me remove my gloves. I wasn't hungry, but I knew I needed to eat. As soon as I took my last bite, the gloves went right back on.

Beep...beep...beep...

The infusion machine was alerting the nurse that the Taxol

portion had been completed. It was time for the Carboplatin.

"How are you feeling? Can I get you anything?"

"I'm OK. Just sleepy."

"Yep, that's from the Benadryl. Take a nap if you can, and if you need to use the restroom, just unplug the infusion machine from the wall and take it with you."

"OK, thank you."

She started the Carboplatin, and I had an immediate reaction. I could feel it entering my body. It felt like it was moving too fast, and I became lightheaded and dizzy. So, the nurse slowed down the speed of the infusion. That did the trick.

When it was time to leave, I got up to go to the bathroom. I felt like I needed to pee so bad. But when I stood up, I felt myself pee a little. The infusion nurse was in the room with me, and I told her what happened and how mortified I was.

"I guess that's just from the chemo, huh?"

"No, it's because you have been holding your pee this whole time. It's OK. You were just nervous."

"Yikes! That's never happened to me before. I guess that tells you just how far outside of my own element I am."

Journal: July 15, 2021

First round of chemo is done. I have a body full of toxins. I'm drinking a ton of water. So much water. H_2Oh my God! They say it's important to stay hydrated and flush out the toxins. So, I spend half the day just peeing it all out. Even my pee is toxic right now. I have to double flush the toilet with the lid down. I literally have poison running through my veins and out of my body. I'm not nauseous, but I feel very weak and sluggish. Yesterday was a lot better. I had enough energy to ride my Peloton and lift weights. Today it was weights only, and even that was tough. I'm going to get a transitional haircut later today because my hair will be falling out soon. Most *likely after next week's chemo. I can't imagine what that's going to be like.*

CHAPTER 7: IMPACT OF CHEMO

"I wouldn't get too comfortable if I were you,"
said Change.

The Chemo Cycle

There's a definite cycle that happens when you're going through chemo, and it dictates a lot of the rhythm. One of the best things I did was to learn the cycle quickly and work within it. Adjusting and adapting my routine and activity to fit the cycle, and not the other way around. The ups, the downs, the good days and bad. Anticipating the nausea and fatigue. Taking anti-nausea medication, which only intensified my fatigue. Dealing with low energy days followed by bursts of energy. Losing my appetite, and then feeling ravenous. Dropping a couple of pounds right after chemo, and then gaining them back just in time for the next round. This was the ebb and flow for the first twelve weeks of chemo. It was a vicious cycle, but it was routine-driven, and I needed that. And there weren't many surprises, because I knew what to expect and when to expect it.

This was especially true when it came to sleep, which played a major role in the cycle. I was always exhausted after chemo, so when I got home, I typically slept for several hours. Sometimes I would even fall asleep in the car as Kenny drove us home.

Sleeping right after chemo was a good thing because the night after chemo would be a sleepless one. I was so jacked up on steroids those nights that sleep was impossible. So instead of tossing and turning in endless frustration, I would stay awake. The kind of awake where you don't even bother turning out the light. I would read, scroll through Facebook and Instagram, watch videos, binge-watch TV shows, and do whatever I could to pass the time until the sun came up.

The next morning, I would feel exhausted and allow myself to take a nap whenever I was ready. Most of the time, I would even workout the day or two after chemo, while my energy level was still up.

But by the third day, everything would start to change. I would feel myself starting to roll downhill uncontrollably. Growing more sluggish by the hour. My body feeling drained and in need of serious rest. My body wanted to sleep. It needed to sleep. It needed a period of inactive recovery. It was involuntary. I would just lie there in my bed, plagued by crippling fatigue, begging to have the strength to get out of bed. It was no use. I had to give in. It was as if every hour that I failed to sleep throughout my entire life had come back to claim its time.

The highs, the lows, and the crashes were all part of an unavoidable cycle. The power comes in learning the cycle and giving in to it, instead of resisting it. Paying close attention to the highs and lows of each day and week. Staying in tune with your energy levels without fighting the natural flow. If you push yourself too hard, your body will let you know, and you can adjust from there. If you can barely hold your head up — and Lord knows there are plenty of days like that — go lie down and take a nap. Give yourself permission. There are no rules. It's all part of the process.

. . .

And then, just when I thought I had the new routine down, boom, it changed again. When I went to the Infusion Center for my ninth round of chemo, my white blood count was too low for chemo that day. So, they gave me a few days to get my numbers up. That's when my chemo day moved from Tuesdays to Fridays. That shifted my sleepless nights and my highs and lows. Some days I wasn't even sure what day it was. And the only movements that made sense were from the bed to the recliner to the sofa to the recliner and back to the bed.

My first round of chemo was on July 13, 2021. My last round was on December 30, 2021. The one thing they all had in common was that semblance of a rhythm. The anxiety the day before each round. The decline. The upswing. The sleepless nights and wakeless days. The fatigue. The nausea. All of it. Each time, without fail.

Hair Is the First to Go

The effects of chemo were immediate, wide-sweeping, and progressive. As time went on, the impact was like the gift that kept on giving, except that it was taking bits and pieces away from me. It would take my hair, my dignity, my self-confidence, my routine, my energy, my physical strength, my endurance, my creativity, my words, my thoughts, my memory, my independence, my youth, my body.

Hair was the first to go, and it happened so early in the process. I didn't get to ease myself into it. And there's no dress rehearsal for bald. Nothing prepares you for losing your hair. One day it's there, and the next day it's gone. I had to accept the inevitable.

I was told I would probably start losing my hair after my second round of chemo. Yep, that's exactly what happened. Just like clockwork. I had just gotten out of the shower and was sitting in my bathroom, about to dry my hair. The more I touched it, the weirder it felt. It didn't even feel like hair. The texture was more like loose, brittle straw. And touching it only made it worse.

I turned on the hairdryer for a few seconds, but it was pointless. I just sat there staring at myself in the mirror. *It's coming out. Stop touching in. Stop looking at it. Just walk away.* The truth is I wanted to scream until there was no scream left in me.

A few hours later, my phone rang. It was the hair salon calling about my wig. Talk about impeccable timing.

"Hi, is this Michelle?"

"Yes, it is."

"Great. I'm calling to let you know your wig is ready whenever you are."

"Ugh. I mean, thank you. The truth is, I'm not sure if I will ever be ready, but it's time. My hair started falling out this morning."

"Oh wow. We can get you in this week if you can come in."

"I have chemo tomorrow, but I could come in the following day if that works."

"Yes, there's an opening at 1 p.m. on Wednesday."

"Great. Please put me down."

I had never wanted anything more and less than I did that wig.

Journal: July 27, 2021

My hair is coming out in clumps now. It was very traumatic this morning in the shower and when I tried to dry my hair. I finally just gave up and left it wet. Nothing but hair in my hairbrush, on my countertop, and on my bathroom floor. Super depressing. I can't even touch it without getting a handful. Now this is real. Very real. Thankfully, my appointment for my wig is Wednesday. They will also be shaving my hair down to about half an inch all over. No one will ever understand what losing hair does to a woman. What it does to this woman.

Before shaving my hair down, I decided to post a video to let everyone know how I was doing and about this traumatic next step. It was the first time I could see the decline in my appearance. I looked terrible. There were strands of misplaced hair streaming across my face and in all the wrong directions. My face was red and puffy, and my eyes looked glassy. If you didn't know better, you might think I had been crying. I had a double set of very pronounced bags underneath both eyes. I was quite the sight.

On the video, I spoke with a hurried tone and the distinct hint of desperation in my voice. I felt rushed to record myself before larger chunks of hair started to fall. It was a bold move to wear a white shirt, given that so much black hair was leaving my head that day.

I know I look like shit, but I only had two hours of sleep last night. I had my pre-chemo steroid yesterday, which keeps me so wired through the night. Anyway, today is the last day you will see my real hair for a while, because it's all coming off and I'm getting a wig. I can either do something similar to my normal look or do something off the wall and outside my comfort zone. There have already been too many changes, so adding one more to the mix seems impossible...

I ended the video by reading a poem I had written a couple of days before. It was a reminder to myself and to others that I was still at least trying to write. Was it my best work? Definitely not. But it was an attempt for me to stay connected to my creative spirit, wherever she may be.

It went like this:

Timing has been known to kill man
It decapitates him
Spilling all the blood
Onto the dry ground below
Without asking permission
It comes and goes
In the dead of night
It steals
And it cashes in
As night falls into darkness
And day vanishes
Like the sun
Just beyond the horizon
And just out of reach
Of the water's edge

I think it was also a reminder that things could be worse. After all, I was losing my hair, not my head. Like most poems, it just wrote itself. I was just the one lucky enough to hold the pen.

Please Pass Me the Scissors

I could feel the dread rushing through me as we entered the doors of the hair salon. Michael went with me. Shortly after I checked in, we were escorted into a private room. Everywhere I looked, I saw mirrors. Everywhere I looked, I saw my reflection.

"Do you think they will let me get the process started? I really feel this compulsion to pick up the scissors and make the first cut."

"I'm sure they will let you do whatever you want to do."

"Good, because I think it would be cathartic, and that's what I need right now."

"I can understand that. I know this is not something you want to be doing today or ever."

"Nope. I still can't believe any of this."

"I know, neither can I. It just doesn't seem fair. Mom wouldn't believe it either."

"I know. I keep trying to imagine what she would say, and I just can't get beyond the disbelief part. She would be in shock, just like us."

Looking over at the sofa, I saw the bright yellow Halston handbag that I brought with me. It was my mom's. Everything about it was her. The color. The buttery soft leather. The small size. The feminine shape. Her love of Halston perfume. The intoxicating scent of patchouli followed her into every room since the early 1980s.

Knock. Knock.

The hairstylist walked into the room holding a Styrofoam head with my wig on it.

"Here it is. What do you think?"

"Um, I think it looks like a lot of hair."

"It is, but we are going to cut and style it based on however you want it to look. Have you thought about the style you would like?"

"Yes, and I really can't deal with anything new. Can you just cut it as similar as possible to the way it looks now?"

"Absolutely. Let me take a look at your layers and see how everything is falling around your face."

"The way it's falling, is that it's falling out. I can show you a few pics from my iPhone so you can see how it looked before all of this."

"OK, great. I will have a look at those after we cut your hair. I will be shaving it down short, like we talked about during your consultation."

"Yep, and I'd like to be the one to make the first cut, if that's OK with you."

"Sure thing. We can go ahead and do that now if you're ready."

"It's now or never. Please pass me the scissors."

I gripped the scissors tightly in my right hand as I reached down and pulled a large section of hair from the top of my head with my left hand. I glanced over at Michael, took a deep breath, and pulled the trigger. For a tiny moment, I had control. Then, I handed the scissors over to the professional to let him do his thing.

Do you know how long it takes to have your head shaved down to a half an inch all the way around? Less than a minute. I'm not sure if that's true, but that's how I remember it. One minute I had hair. The next, it was gone.

. . .

As Michael and I left the hair salon together, I turned to him and suggested that he shave his head as a gesture of support and solidarity. And, like all brothers, he said *no!* That's OK. I didn't really want or need that from him or anyone. I'm not a believer in the concept of misery loves company. I didn't envy his hair or his health. Instead, I thanked God he wasn't going through this. But he was going through this, just like Kenny was.

Journal: July 31, 2021

My hair is gone. On Wednesday, I shaved it down to a buzz cut. Not me exactly, but the guy at the wig place. The wig looks just like my hair, but it's just too much to wear all day, every day. It's heavy and hot. Every time I see myself in the mirror, I want to cry or scream or both. I don't love my nearly bald head. And it's hard to sleep at night. Nothing feels comfortable. I've invested in a couple of hats, but nothing feels normal. We have strayed a long way from normal.

I'm a Hat Person

I decided to do a wig reveal video and post it on Facebook. And fortunately, everyone was complimentary and said all the right things.

But I knew the truth. When the wig comes off and I'm staring at myself in the mirror, the horror is undeniable. To see your reflection with little to no hair is not something you ever really get used to. I know hair is a small price to pay when you're fighting for your life, but that doesn't make it any less traumatic.

So, when you are a woman faced with complete hair loss, one of the questions you ask yourself is: *Am I a wig person, or a hat person, or a scarf person, or a bald person?* I was sure I wanted a wig right off the bat. I thought how I looked was something I could control. That wig was beautiful, natural, human hair, and it look almost identical to my style. You couldn't have asked for a better wig.

But I hated it. I only wore it about ten times, and each time I felt self-conscious about it. I was sure people could tell. It made me feel like a fraud. Besides that, it was hot, heavy, and uncomfortable. So, I realized I was not a wig person. It turns out that I was a hat person.

And, as I write this, I am beyond blessed and thankful to say that I am once again a hair person.

The Good, the Bad, the Bald

There were good days, and there were bad days. I wanted to share the honesty of all the moments. Good moments and bad ones. And all of them featured the bald moments, as my head quickly transformed from a buzz cut to bald. There was nowhere to hide. It was raw. It was real. And it never failed to surprise and shock. There it was — my bald head. I could cover it with wigs and hats, but underneath was the truth.

Once I lost my hair, I wore a hat for all photos and outings. I never took any bald photos, even for me. That wasn't an image I wanted to capture for all eternity. I didn't want to commit it to memory or immortalize it. I never felt bald and beautiful, I just felt bald.

That's why it's so surprising, even now, that I allowed people to see me at my worst. I just kept thinking, *it is what it is, and you can't completely hide it.* It's not like a pimple you can cover with make-up, or an extra five pounds you can hide under a big shirt or jacket.

Nonetheless, I wanted to document my journey. All of it. The good, the bad, the bald. Initially, I thought I was pulling back the curtain to give people a peek at what I was going through, but it became much more than that. It became a combined act of courage and vulnerability that was met with deep empathy and encouragement. And the outpouring of love and support I received from my family and friends near and far, let me know I wasn't in this alone. No matter how lonely and isolating it would become, I was able to share and connect with people on a whole new level. And I loved that.

The Camera Doesn't Lie

The change in my appearance became progressively worse. I

would often gasp in disbelief when I played back my videos. And I always used the first take, because I didn't want them to be perfect and polished. It was supposed to be real, in-the-moment, authentic snippets captured on video. Yes, I had a bald head lurking underneath my hat. I had an eyelash or two, zero eyebrows except for the ones I penciled in, puffy eyes and cheeks, a pale complexion, and glassy eyes. Yep, that was me now.

The camera doesn't lie, and neither does the mirror. Both shined a spotlight on the stark reality of the situation and my deteriorating appearance. Day in and day out, there was no escape.

In my videos, there was no hiding my bald head, even with baseball caps and hats. The peach fuzz was always visible on the sides. I could also see the changes on my face and in my eyes. The color was drained from my cheeks, and my almond-shaped eyes looked drawn and squinty.

I studied my photos and my videos, and relentlessly compared them with the healthy me. *Thank you, Facebook for the memories, not!* They were daily reminders of how I used to look just a short time ago. I would think, *hard to believe that was only a year ago or two years ago. Look at me and how young and fit I look. That was a good hair day and look at how bright my eyes are. Look at those long eyelashes.*

Chemo Brain

Chemo brain. That's what they call it. I started to experience it right after my second round. I realized I wasn't firing on all cylinders. I could feel that I was off. Struggling to find the right words. There was this sense of fogginess when I spoke. I was stuck in my head, combing through my dictionary for the right words. Hunting them down. Trying to remember. Getting lost in my own words mid-sentence. The simplest of words. Just gone. It was like they were being kept prisoner in a dark room without food or water.

Sometimes the elusive word was so ordinary, that I was embarrassed for having misplaced it. One time it was *sunburn.*

How do you lose *sunburn*? The word was just out of reach. Like when you try to remember a dream you had the night before, and you chase it as it wanders further and further away. The harder you try to catch it, the more it drifts away, until it finally disappears forever.

Meanwhile, there I was. Stuck in mid-sentence. Purgatory. Forced to listen to my own ramblings. I would often veer off in a new direction just to speak the words that came more easily. It was difficult for me to hear, so I can only imagine how it must have felt to those who were forced to listen.

Chemo brain also took over my hand every time I picked up a pen. I could see the deterioration of my cohesive thoughts on paper, combined with misspellings, repeating lines and sentences, and the most unpleasant thing of all — words crossed out completely. It was relentless.

At the height of my chemo brain, I was forced to do the impossible. I had to renew my real estate broker's license. That meant taking online mandatory continuing education classes and passing exams. There was a lot riding on it, so I couldn't screw up. I gave myself plenty of time, took it slow, and powered through. There was no other way.

Looking back, taking those classes, and passing those exams was nothing short of amazing, given my mental and physical state. It was like that recurring dream where you have a test, but you haven't been to school all semester. I wasn't naked in this dream, but I was bald and without a hat, so it was similar.

Phone calls were another thing that became more difficult as time went on. I felt this increasing need to build myself up before making an ordinary call. My confidence had plummeted right along with my energy level. So, I didn't want to talk to anyone unless I really felt up to the task. Sometimes I would sit there unable to place a call. Feeling paralyzed. Making calls used to be the easy part. Suddenly, there were no easy parts. It was all hard.

Creativity

Where does your creativity go when you are unable to give it life? Does it move on to someone else, or hibernate until the long winter has ended? Does it simply wait for you, or grow tired of the separation? You never know for sure, but sometimes it's the risk you are forced to take.

Not only was the poison killing my cancer, but it was also killing my creativity. It was waging war on the very essence of what makes me, me. *Dear God, please let this be temporary.* I prayed about that too. That this thing — this living, breathing organism that has lived within me since my childhood — wouldn't give up on me. That it would wait patiently for me and return to me. And that I wouldn't let it down.

Soon, everything I wrote felt flat and forced, but I kept doing it anyway. At least I could enjoy the feeling of the pen in my hand and my movements across the empty page. It was a practice. A routine. But there were days when the pen didn't even feel right in my hand. Like I was holding something that didn't want to be held. It was trying to pry my fingers open and set itself free.

Surrounded by Books

I surrounded myself with books. This was nothing new. As a writer, I have a great appreciation for books and have amassed quite a collection. And there is something magical about having certain books within reach when you need a little inspiration. The more I struggled to find my own words, the more I wanted to surround myself with the words of others. It was comforting. It reminded me that there is always inspiration. Sometimes, you just have to know where to look for it.

And after my diagnosis, I knew just where to look. Next to me, on the upper right corner of my desk sits a pile of books I have carefully chosen for inspiration. Some books are staples, while others rotate in and out of the pile based on what I need the most at any given moment. I need to keep these books within easy reach. They keep me connected to my creative world.

After my diagnosis and throughout my *journey*, the pile of books continued to grow. I kept needing more. And the more I struggled to create, the more I reached for that pile. There was an intrinsic need to take a deeper dive and peruse the pages in search of new meaning and inspiration. Surrounded by books, hoping the words would just fall out and land all over me.

Taste Buds

I already ate a healthy diet, but there were some changes I had to make. Namely, I was put on a high-protein diet because it was important for me to increase my protein intake while going through chemo. Protein is needed to repair body tissue, help fight infection, and to keep the immune system healthy.

I had to start eating breakfast too. That wasn't easy, because I spent most of my life skipping breakfast. So, breakfast became a new staple in my morning routine.

Apart from that, my diet was similar to the pregnancy diet. I wasn't supposed to eat undercooked or raw meat. No more medium rare steaks. No sushi. I was also discouraged from eating raw fruits and vegetables, especially if they were prepared in a restaurant. Improper washing of fruits and vegetables and the personal hygiene of those preparing them was not worth the risk. So, I followed the rules.

My taste buds also changed several times during treatment. So, I learned to roll with that too. Sometimes the only thing I wanted to eat was the most bland meal imaginable. Maybe a chicken breast with a little bit of salt and pepper, some green peas, and a baked potato. Other times, the more flavorful, the better. Those were the nights when Kenny would order dinner from our favorite Indian restaurant. I devoured lamb vindaloo that was so spicy it made my eyes water.

Probably the most surprising part was that I drank very little coffee throughout my treatment. It just didn't taste right. And my penchant for sweets was lacking too. There was the occasional chocolate chip cookie, and a bowl of ice cream here and there, but that was about it.

Instead, I craved the salty tartness of salad. Not just any salad — *the* salad. My Maw-Maw Pearl's salad. The simple concoction of extra virgin olive oil, white vinegar, salt, pepper, and a few pinches of sugar tossed into a waiting bowl of sliced baby cucumber, red bell pepper, purple onion, cherry tomatoes, and radishes. Just the thought of it made my mouth water. All I had to do was close my eyes, and suddenly I was standing in her kitchen — my favorite place on earth. The strong fragrant aroma of her famous fried chicken, lingering there in all its glory. She always let me taste one of the delicious slices of perfectly marinated cucumber. The taste of my childhood. She would clasp her fingers around my shoulder and say: *Go ahead. Have one more, but that's it until supper.*

. . .

Kenny, Michael, and Joanne took me to a local cafeteria a few times while I was going through chemo. That was a good choice because of the wide variety of selections.

There is one time that sticks out to me. I had just placed my napkin and silverware roll on my tray. That's when I saw it — fried chicken. It looked so delicious I could almost taste it.

I turned to Kenny and said, "I think I'm going to have the fried chicken."

"Alright! You should definitely have the fried chicken. You need to have whatever sounds good to you, because you need to eat."

Then the lady behind the counter asked me what I would like. I opened my mouth to say *fried chicken*, but my mouth said *roast beef.* The idea of fried chicken seemed too self-indulgent. Like a guilty pleasure that was forbidden. So, I had the roast beef, and it was delicious. But I still regret that moment to this day. I should have said the right words. I should have said *fried chicken.*

Signal of Strength

It wasn't always easy, but I did my best. I didn't want to look sick and frail and weak. Not at the beginning, not in the middle, and certainly not at the end. Instead, I wanted to show that I was strong, even when I could barely hold my head up. I wanted and hoped to inspire strength in others. Even when I wasn't feeling it. Especially then, because it helped me shut down my inner voice. To silence it. To fake it if I had to.

Even with all the changes, I wanted to portray myself as a signal of strength. Not just for those around me and those looking in, but also for myself. Every time I looked in the mirror, I wanted to still be able to find that strong woman I knew I was. She was sometimes a little hidden from me, but I could squint my eyes and still find her.

So, a few weeks before I started losing my hair, I shot that image I saw of myself. I was wearing my mom's oversized white Ray-bans, flexing my muscles, and smiling from ear to ear. This was my social media profile picture for months. I thought it sent the right message to the world. It laughed in the face of cancer. It gave me power, while allowing me to feel like I was channeling my mom. It said, *I'm strong, I'm fierce, I'm a fighter, and I've got this.*

People said I was a warrior. An inspiration. And that cancer didn't have a chance against me. So, that was the image I wanted to showcase. This strong version of myself with a full head of hair. Showing cancer who's boss. This positive, smiling creature was a surprise, especially to me.

CHAPTER 8: ACCEPTING HELP

---

*I am definitely a swimmer, but that doesn't mean I
don't sometimes need a life jacket.*

Kenny

I began shooting short videos from the Infusion Center and
posting them each week to let everyone know how I was doing.
Each time, Kenny would stand silently next to my chemo chair,
smiling awkwardly into the camera. Being front and center was
never his thing, but he agreed to stand next to me. His face had
become as familiar as my own on those videos.

Before long, people were leaving comments on my Facebook
posts asking to hear from Kenny. So, I promised he would speak
on video soon. I didn't realize how much he had considered it,
until the moment of truth.

One morning from the infusion chair, I hit the record button,
asked Kenny to talk about what things were like from his
perspective, and he famously declared his role.

> *I've been thinking about what to say, and wondering why
> y'all are so anxious to hear from me, and this thought
> occurred. Whenever you see a visually impaired person
> walking around, and they have a service animal, people
> always want to pay attention to the service animal. And
> they're told, don't pet the service animal. I think in this
> situation, I am Michelle's service animal.*
>
> *Don't think that's a bad thing, because I think dogs
> might be the highest form of life on this planet. So, my
> job is to do the things for Michelle that she can't do for
> herself, and more importantly, to enable her to do the*

83

things she can do. It's really that simple.

And just like that, a star was born. The comments started pouring in. He was so sweet and humble in his soft-spoken tone. His words were genuine, straight from the heart. I knew he was nervous, but he had taken this so seriously as to have something prepared and ready to go.

We all need a support animal, and Kenny designated himself as mine. This wasn't unique to me having cancer; he has always been my greatest supporter. Ever indulgent, always saying yes.

He had called it perfectly. He was my service animal, but more importantly, he was my rock. Completely unflappable no matter what was thrown my way. The truth is, we never really talked about how everything affected him. There were times when I read the look of concern on his face. I could see the tinge of fear, but he did his best to hide it from me. Suddenly, all those domestic arguments pretty much fell away. They just didn't matter anymore. We had to focus on the big stuff, and there was no shortage of big stuff. He was scared of losing me, and I was scared of leaving him.

I once read that in marriage, sometimes you are the garden, and sometimes you are the gardener. Right then, I was the garden, which was unusual for me. I'm a much better gardener. But there was no one I'd rather have looking after me than Kenny — my master gardener.

After thirty-five years of marriage, we had lived our vows. *For better or worse. In sickness and in health.* No matter what life throws at us, we are in it together forever. Tied and bound. Soul mates. Cell mates. Garden and gardener. Opposites in every way. Completely different upbringings and backgrounds. It was nothing short of a miracle that our paths ever crossed at all. A wonder for the ages. Fate is a beautiful thing. *Bashert.* Meant to be.

He later said to me, "My role is really to fall in to whatever your rhythm is, and to fill in where needed."

"That's like ghost notes in drumming. Ghost notes are the softer notes played on the snare drum in between accented beats.

They make a groove more interesting."

"Yep, it's exactly like that."

. . .

We were fortunate that his employer allowed him the flexibility to work from home most of the time, and to be with me for every appointment. And on days when I was in bed, he worked wonders — he juggled my needs, work, dogs, and sometimes laundry. It was a lot, but it's what you do.

There were also new rules around everyday things. There was silence when silence was what I needed. There were times when I couldn't even bear the low volumed whisper of a single word. I needed only to hear my own breath and to meditate on the miracle of that. It's the simplest thing you can do to prove you're still alive. Most of the time, Kenny understood and would honor my wish. Other times, he spoke anyway, not understanding how loud it already was in my head. He couldn't help himself, but he didn't want to argue either. Not now, and maybe never again.

People Will Surprise You

People will surprise you. This is true from the moment they hear that you have cancer, throughout your treatment, surgeries, and even long past the point when you have healed. They will surprise you in good ways and bad. People who I least expected to show up for me at all, showed up in the most spectacular ways imaginable. Meanwhile, some of the people I expected to show up in the biggest ways, were spectacularly absent. They only showed up in small drips, if at all.

The support and encouragement I received was nonstop. The gifts, the meals, the gift cards, the messages, the texts, and the phone calls. So many comforting items continuously arrived at my doorstep. They included a New Orleans Doberge cake, a tin of Louisiana pecans, chocolates, cookies, LSU pillows, blankets, T-shirts, books, journals, orchids, hats, scented candles, bandanas, and bracelets. The list goes on and on. And my heart was indeed full.

. . .

Sometimes, I even received unexpected advice from unexpected people. Like the phone call I had with my uncle, my mom's only brother. We were not close. In fact, we hadn't seen each other in twenty years, but we had spoken on the phone a few times since my mom's death. So, I called him one night to let him know about my diagnosis. I just thought he should know. I wasn't expecting anything, much less advice, but it turned out to be the best advice he could have given me.

"So much has happened in such a short time, between losing my mom and now getting cancer. It's a lot for one person to deal with, and I'm struggling."

"Try to come to grips with what has happened, understand it, get through it, and then leave it behind you and live your life," he said.

So simple. So profound. And spot on.

I didn't know it at the time, but that would be our last conversation. He has since passed, so this was the last piece of advice he ever gave me. Apart from some photographs, it's everything I have of him. But those words were a gift. They are now legacy.

Max & Stella

Max and Stella — my real support animals. My beloved English Bulldogs.

They say animals know when you're sick. They can sense it or smell it, or somehow just know. This was the case with Max and Stella. The first thing I noticed was that Max stopped sitting on my lap. This happened right away. He knew. We are so connected and have been since the moment we first laid eyes on each other. It was like he was afraid to sit on my lap in case it might hurt me.

That made me sad, because there is something very intimate about your dog wanting to be that close to you.

Stella picked up on it too. She wasn't one to sit on my lap, but she liked to sit close. I think she realized I was sick before Max did. I can't explain it, but I saw something in her eyes when she looked at me. And she saw the confirmation in my eyes when I looked back at her. She became a little gentler around me. She was a bit cuddlier too. It was sweet and sad at the same time.

They provided an extra layer of love and comfort at all the right times. They sat next to me on the sofa, and watched closely every time I crossed the room. Their eyes followed me up and down the stairs. And whenever I reappeared after being stuck in the bed for a while, they were excited to see me again. *There she is! There's our mom!*

Asking for Help

It's hard for me to admit to needing anything, least of all help. And asking for help? Well, that's out of the question. But everyone was asking the same thing: *What can I do to help you?* They wanted to do something, anything, but they weren't sure what. People were asking Michael the same question.

So, he came up with a solution.

"What if I start a meal train for you so you don't have to think about what's for dinner every night? I know you like to cook, but it's going to get harder for you now, so why not take some of the burden off you and Kenny?"

"No way! People will think I can't feed myself, or even worse, that I can't afford it."

"It's not like that at all. People just want to do something to help you and make you more comfortable."

"But it feels like a financial contribution, and that's the last thing I want anyone thinking."

"People won't think that. They just want to know what they can do to help. Besides, it wouldn't come from you; it would be from me. Why don't we try it for a little while."

"I don't know. Like how long?"

"A month or two? I can set it up, and we can see how it goes."

"I guess so, but it feels embarrassing."

"Trust me, it's not."

That night Michael set it up and posted the information on his Facebook page. Within forty-eight hours, people had signed up to bring or have dinner delivered to us for the next eight weeks. I couldn't believe it. And once all the dates were filled on the calendar, people continued to send gift cards and randomly drop off meals and other goodies for the next several months. It was incredible.

Still, I didn't want to be that person, the one who asks for help. It just wasn't in my DNA. But guess what? Cancer don't care about that either. Giving into Michael and the meal train was one of the smartest decisions I could have made. I was in no shape to cook every night, and Kenny wasn't exactly a chef. His entire cooking repertoire consisted of: eggs, grits, toast, canned soup, and grilled cheese.

Some years ago, I wrote: *Plans sometimes capsize. It's up to you to be a swimmer.* I had to remind myself that although I was a strong swimmer, on occasion, I needed someone to toss me a life jacket.

The meal train was a way of letting people help me, while making life a little easier for me and Kenny. I realize that now. It was about letting others do the things for me that I couldn't do for myself, as Kenny had so eloquently stated.

When you don't have enough strength on the outside, you have to rely on your strength on the inside. And when you don't have enough of your own strength on the inside, you must rely again on strength from the outside in terms of other people.

You might wake up some mornings asking yourself, *do I have it in me? Do I have the fight in me today?* And the answer has to be a resounding *yes,* every damn time. And if you don't know if you can do it today, then let others do the heavy lifting for you. Lean in when you need to lean in and rise up when you are able to rise up.

. . .

Asking for help takes many different forms. There are the traditional ones, like therapy, and there are the ones no one ever sees and rarely talks about. Like reading old comments and text messages, or looking for an inspirational message or guidance within books, or videos, or even prayers to God. Sometimes I seek help through meditation, or on my Peloton, or from sitting on the sofa with Max, his paw in my hand. Or I might write about it, or find a poem lurking around in my head, waiting to be born.

Asking for help, that's not something that comes easily for me. There's this voice in my head that says, *asking for help is admitting weakness.* But I couldn't be more wrong. It means that I recognize my limitations and need to engage my resources.

It usually takes me a little while to realize when a situation is beyond me and requires the help or intervention of others. I'm not sure why I'm that way, but I am. This is what makes your tribe — your support system — so invaluable. People can't help you if you don't reach out and share your concerns with them. You have to let them know how you're feeling. Let them know how they can help you.

And although we have these wonderful people in our lives who love and support us, sometimes it helps to wander a little further outside of our immediate circles for advice or to talk. In my case, I wanted to protect the emotions of the people around me. At times, I even downplayed how I was feeling. I didn't want anyone to worry about me any more than they already did.

CHAPTER 9: FINDING A NEW RHYTHM

---

*Nothing inhibits the flow of thought more than the
disruption of rhythm.*

Rhythm

I've heard people say cancer is a full-time job. Boy, they weren't
kidding. Between all the doctors' appointments and phone calls,
the chemo cycle, the ups and downs, there was little time for
anything else. Cancer isn't something you can compartmentalize.
It's cancer, for fuck sake. All day, every day. No breaks. It
requires everything you have. Every minute of every day. There
is nothing else. Only this. Only cancer.

So, I had to make some changes and adjustments to my
routine, all of which were immediate. I hated that. I'm such a
routine-driven person, and I've always treated my routine as
something sacred to be rigidly followed. But I had to deal with all
this new stuff, while trying to hold on to some of my old stuff.
That threw my entire rhythm off.

For me, it all comes down to rhythm. When your rhythm is
off, everything is off. You're out of step with your life and the
rest of the world. You're offbeat and singing out of tune. There's
no flow. Only stops and starts, and ups and downs, and forwards
and backwards. It's a very odd time signature.

That's tough for me as a 4/4 kind of drummer who needs to
hear the backbeat on two and four. There's a symmetry to that,
and it makes sense to me. But now, there was this disruption to
my carefully crafted rhythm. Like when my mom died, and
everything came to a grinding halt. There I was, slamming on the
brakes again. Trying to catch my breath. Trying to put one
wobbly foot in front of the other. I would have to learn to move
my body to a new rhythm. One that went against my natural flow.

Rhythm is also about how our everyday movement is driven

by repeated routines and patterns. That underlying beat we hear and follow. The underlying organization and structure. It requires consistency, without disruption. Constant flow, without friction. Rhythm is a grounding force, where everything is in agreement and is understood. The time signature. The tempo. All of it. It keeps me on course and guides me through my morning, afternoon, and nighttime rituals. It rises and falls with every breath. It pauses and resumes in melodic fashion. It's the very beating of my heart. The ticking of my internal clock. It's the pulse. The pulse of everything.

I had mastered my old rhythm. It was my routine, chock-full of daily rituals and reminders. It was smooth and easy to execute. *Keep moving. Work out six days a week. Ride the Peloton every other day. Lift weights. Walk every afternoon that it doesn't rain. Run a little. Throw some yoga into the mix. Meditate. Silence the outside noise as much as possible. Stay away from toxic people and situations. Be open to creative musings. Write every day. Wear a uniform — T-shirt, jeans, and sneakers. Walk the dogs. Maintain a healthy weight. Fuel my body. Don't eat processed foods. Don't drink alcohol. Keep pushing yourself harder. Treat your body like a temple.* So, the idea of changing this well-oiled machine was a difficult one.

Change has never come easy for me. Even the smallest change can throw me into a tailspin. And now there was this major disruption taking place, threatening everything I had worked so hard to build and maintain. Like an implosion, blowing out all my windows. Dust and debris as far as the eyes could see.

I was powerless, and I had to learn to exist within this new rhythm. It was one I had no control over, so I had to work with what I had. And in the process, I learned a new concept: *flexibility*.

So, I'm not sure if you find a new rhythm or if a new rhythm finds you. Either way, you have no choice. Control what you can and give in to the rest.

Day of Chemo

I always woke up feeling grumpy on the day of chemo. It wasn't any wonder. I rarely slept the night before, consumed by racing thoughts that wouldn't settle down. I would toss and turn and check my iPhone all night to see what time it was. To see how many hours until I had to get up. And, despite knowing the cycle, I was never ready to have chemo again. Never ready repeat the cycle.

It didn't help that I am not a morning person. That means I don't like to talk or have anyone talk to me for at least an hour after waking up. Kenny understood and kept the chatter to a minimum.

Every chemo day started out the same. Roll out of bed, go to the bathroom, brush my teeth, get on the Peloton, take a shower, put my make-up on, and get dressed.

Most people wouldn't have bothered with make-up, but that's not how my mom raised me. I never left the house without it. I would never consider it. I was hard-wired that way. I can still hear my mom's soft, yet firm voice. *Look good on the outside and you will feel better on the inside.* And so, I went to chemo dressed to kill — dressed to kill cancer.

. . .

As soon as I was dressed, I headed downstairs, where Kenny was waiting for me. We had a ritual. I would make my breakfast, which was always Greek yogurt with a banana or blueberries, and he would put the Lidocaine cream on my port and cover it with plastic wrap. This was helpful in numbing the area where my port would be accessed for chemo. He would ask me how I was feeling or something equally inoffensive, and I would feel like I could snap. But he took whatever verbal abuse I spewed his way. It was OK. He understood.

Chemo time was always at 10 a.m. That meant pulling out of the driveway at exactly 9 a.m. You could set a clock by me. There was no way I was ever going to deviate from that schedule. We would take my car, and I would drive us to the hospital. I wouldn't be able to drive us home, but I could at least get us there.

As soon as the car cleared our garage, we had another ritual. Kenny would look at me and reach for my hand.

"Hey Michelle, you know what?"

"No, what?"

"Today's going to be a good day."

"How do you know?"

"Trust me. I just know."

I was filled with so much dread, and my anxiety was at level ten. But, when Kenny spoke those words: *today's going to be a good day*, I believed him.

Few other words were spoken in the car. I only had the capacity to focus on getting us there. The softness of his palm pressing against the back of my hand as we drove.

Once we arrived at the hospital, the routine was always the same. Park in the garage. Walk through the hospital grounds in silence, with me leading the way several feet ahead of Kenny. I was always ready to get there, get started, and check another round of chemo off the list.

Then we walked inside the Infusion Center together. I checked in, got my wristband, got weighed, and was escorted to my tiny room. My private cave behind the sliding door and drawn curtain. I removed my iPhone, reading glasses, and Altoids from my purse and placed them on the tray connected to the chemo chair. I reclined the chair and turned on the seat heater. It was always freezing in there. Kenny would sit in the small chair to my right because the infusion machine was on my left.

From there, it was boom, boom, boom. My vitals were checked, my port was accessed and flushed with saline, and my blood was drawn and sent to the lab. Then I would record a quick video and post it to Facebook, followed by Kenny walking out of the room in search of coffee. That's when I would turn on the TV, wait for the lab results, and everything else that followed.

As soon as the chemo was started, I would feel my eyes grow heavier, as my gaze dashed between Kenny and the TV. He would watch me struggle to keep my eyes open. He would wink at me and say, "Don't fight it. Close your eyes and go to sleep."

I would feel myself drifting in and out of sleep as the chemo bag emptied itself into my veins.

I was often awakened by the sound of the beeping infusion machine announcing the end of another round.

The rest was easy. My port was flushed, we went home, and I crashed in the bed.

It helped to fall into the rhythm. To follow the same process and monotonous routine. I knew what to expect, so there wasn't that initial fear of the unknown.

A Sliver of Normalcy

Part of accepting the new rhythm was the ability to stay connected to parts of the old one. It's about finding a sliver of normalcy amid the disruption. For me, nothing connected me more to my old routine than my Peloton. I wasn't willing to stop under any circumstances, no matter how rough it became. Throughout my treatment, I managed to get in a total of forty-two Peloton rides.

I wanted to sweat those toxins out of my bloodstream. To have sweat dripping down my face was preferable to tears. It was the closest I came to crying. There's a very emotional, meditative aspect to working out, and I desperately needed that too.

My rationale was simple: *My Peloton saved me once, and I needed it to save me again.* And it did. Those pre-chemo rides became progressively more difficult, especially near the end, but I did them anyway. I told myself that all wasn't bad or lost as long as I could do this. It was a mandate from myself. A gentle push. *You can do this. You will do this, and you will smile. It's going to get harder, but that's OK. You must do it anyway.*

Walking was another carryover from my old routine. I continued my walks through the neighborhood, complete with live videos encouraging others to walk and exercise. To take care of their bodies and remain diligent about any unusual changes that could warrant a visit to the doctor.

And when I was unable to walk or ride my Peloton or hardly

move at all, I asked others to do it for me. Feeling supported is a two-way street. Encouragement gives life to encouragement.

Please walk with me and for me. You're not just part of the journey; you're a necessary part of the healing. The emotional and physical healing. Just get out and walk and breathe some fresh air. Keep your legs moving and do something that feels normal to you. Something that you control. Heed my warning. You never know what's around the next corner and coming for you. I sure didn't, and I don't know what's around the next one either. None of us do. Make every moment count. Make every day count. Make every breath count. And just keep moving forward.

. . .

Working out was also an essential strategy for keeping my anxiety at bay. Or at least pausing it for a few minutes. There were days when my anxiety felt like a rising river with flood waters coming up over the banks. Everything seemed out of control. But working out shifted my focus. It allowed me to take a short sabbatical from my worry. Working out felt normal. Riding my Peloton felt normal. And walking felt normal, so I wanted to hold on to those things for dear life.

Productivity

Productivity. That feeling you should be doing something worthwhile with your time, but you just don't have it in you. Creatively bankrupt. Upset by your own inactivity. Energy-crushing fatigue taking over your entire body. Showing no mercy.

Productivity. For me, the word itself was more of a distraction than anything else. It meant that I spent my day doing something deliberate. Something worthy and with intention.

One afternoon, I spent hours in my office using my label maker. I labeled every notebook, journal, and planner. On the surface, this was a seemingly unnecessary task, but it was surprisingly satisfying. There I was, manically trying out different fonts and styles, as if this was serious, critical work that required precise attention to detail. Yet, it passed the time, so it felt like a win. I had forced myself to stay in my office and get something done. Complete a project. Have a sense of accomplishment.

Before long, forcing myself to stay in my office had become my go-to move. My hack for staying out of my bed. It fooled everyone, even me. I would just sit there at my desk letting idol hours pass by. I would scroll through websites, or write in my journal, or read inspirational passages from the books on my desk, or look at old photos and videos, or call a friend, or just stare out the window. It didn't matter. The only thing that mattered was that I stayed there.

It wasn't easy, but it worked. I would sit there in my office, at my desk, and hide away from the world, my illness, and myself. It was a successful strategy, and I practiced it like an art. *Let the clock tick and take you from one minute to the next. One hour to the next. You can do this. All you have to do is sit here until you can't sit here anymore.*

Some days it was enough to just sit there and make To-Do lists. It was even cathartic. *Pay Visa bill, make vet appointment, order printer cartridges, buy toothpaste, make bank deposit, refill prescriptions, research protein powders, renew flood insurance policy.*

My lists kept me grounded in the everyday. In the mundane minutia of life. It allowed me to steady my thoughts and focus on something else. Anything else.

My planner had become a dumping ground for my endless array of medical appointments. So, it was a nice diversion to fill a few pages with tasks unrelated to and disconnected from this thing — this dominant thing — that ruled over every aspect of my life. I could pretend, at least on paper, that I had all these other things to do. Reminders of the real world.

Monday Morning Video Calls

I didn't let go of work completely. And fortunately, one of my clients didn't let go of me completely either. Thank goodness, because I needed to feel useful. To have a purpose outside of what was going on in my body and in my house. It was just enough work, without the pressure of a real job. In fact, there was no pressure at all. No stress. No anxiety. I was able to work at my own pace and on my own terms, based solely on how I was feeling and what I was physically and mentally able to do. But there was a kicker, and it was a big one.

Every other Monday morning, I was invited to attend and participate in their team meetings. Not in person, but by video. So, my image was projected onto the big screen in their conference room. Being bald and having biweekly 9 a.m. video calls was not ideal, but it gave me a reason to get out of bed and make myself presentable. It kept me from pulling the covers up over my head and calling it a day. Those video calls, though somewhat embarrassing, gave me a sense of temporary purpose. Looking back, it was brave, given the state of me.

The Slow Down

Life slowed down in a way that was completely unfamiliar. I slowed down in a way that scared me. I felt the weight of every single day. Some days were much heavier than others. And there was a silence. A quiet. A loneliness that comes both from within and without. And I was both more and less of myself. My sense of self-reliance was peeling back and revealing my need for assistance. A fear that rose and fell with each breath. An undeniable urgency that determined the course of action. My life instantly became that course of action. A rigid agenda to be followed to the letter. A series of appointments, instructions, and obstacles, all carefully strung together just for me. Go here. Go there. Do this. Do that. Don't do that. And don't look ahead too far. Stay in the moment. This moment. Breathe. Trust us. Trust the process. Trust yourself. And the sun will rise and set again tomorrow.

I Just Want to Get Out of Bed

The fourth and fifth days after chemo were the roughest in terms of side effects. This was part of the rhythm too. The nausea and fatigue really got to me. There were many days when all I wanted was to get out of bed. You'd think that would have been so easy. Just sit up, swing your legs around, and get off the bed. But no, I couldn't do it. It was impossible. I had the will, but I didn't have an ounce of strength. I couldn't even lift my head off the pillow. I would just lie there in the fetal position with two pillows underneath my head and one between my knees. I pleaded for the strength to get out of bed. It was agonizing.

I would listen intently for Kenny's footsteps. He had made a habit of checking on me several times a day. I always felt a little relieved and less alone when I could hear him coming. His heavy shoes pounding against the wooden stairs. I would silently count each step as he climbed. One, two, three, four…nineteen.

He would turn the corner into our bedroom and quietly walk over to the bed, stretching his neck out to see if I was asleep.

"It's OK, I'm awake."

"I wasn't sure. I came up here about an hour ago, and you were sacked. How are you feeling?"

"Like shit."

"What's bothering you the most?"

"I'm nauseous, I have a splitting headache, and I hate lying in bed all day. I've been sleeping so much, yet I feel exhausted."

"I'm sorry. Is there something I can get you or something I can do for you?"

"No, not really. I just want to get up and get out of this bed. I'm tired of sleeping and I'm tired of doing nothing."

"I know, but it's the best thing you can do right now. Your body needs to rest, so just let it rest."

"I've been in this bed too long. I can't take it anymore."

"Just remember that this isn't forever. You are doing great. Everything is working just like it's supposed to, and you will get through this. Get some rest, and I will come back and check on you a little later."

"OK. I guess."

"If you need me sooner, just text me."

While his words were encouraging, all I really wanted to do was lift my limp body out of the bed. Was that too much to ask? I've never experienced that level of fatigue before. Even with a hangover, you are glad to be in bed all day if that's what it takes. This was different. My body was much weaker than my brain. It just refused to function properly.

Why Bother?

Why bother? Why bother, indeed! There will be many days when you just want to stay in bed with the covers pulled up over your head. Sometimes that's because it really is all you can manage. You're tired, fatigued, exhausted, nauseous. So, you find yourself thinking, *what's the point?* Why bother getting out of bed? Why bother getting up and taking a shower and getting dressed? Why bother with my day or my routine?

These feelings are normal. And giving in to them would be the easy thing to do. But try to resist. Your real strength lies in your ability to do the hard stuff. And that means not giving in to the voices in your own head. You have to get out of your own way.

Yes, there will be days when the sheer energy it takes to get out of bed will feel overwhelming and even like a dramatic feat. That's the point. Do the hard stuff. Put in the work. Do tough things. It will give you much-needed strength on your weakest days. Just like the days when I would sit in my office all afternoon, resisting the urge to take a nap. I knew it was keeping me out of bed. Mind over matter. So, I continually forced myself, day after grueling day, *when I could*. That's the important part — *when I could*.

I also listened to my body and knew that some days this was going to be impossible. It's not just mind over matter. Yes, I know I'm contradicting myself, but in many ways, that's also the point. It's just what happens. Try to control what you can and let the rest go. It's part of the ironic dichotomy of the situation.

Sitting in my office, no matter how awful I felt, gave me power. It gave me strength and control over the demons that wanted free range over my thoughts. I didn't give in. I couldn't give in.

Why bother, you ask? Why bother, indeed!

CHAPTER 10: EMOTIONAL ROLLER COASTER

Under the cover of darkness, there is a riptide of emotion waiting to erupt.

Emotions

My emotions ran wild from the moment I was lying on the hospital bed reading the radiologist's face as she read my ultrasound. Some days my emotions felt like they were swinging from a chandelier. Other days my emotions felt like they were lying face down, motionless in a ditch. It ran the full gamut.

The most negative emotions were locked away on the inside, while the positive ones were dancing around unfettered on the outside. I tried hard to keep the negative thoughts out of my head, but they had nowhere else to go. Some days they were more in check than others. I desperately wanted to keep it all positive, which meant sometimes faking it for everyone around me, including myself. Each day, each event, each appointment, each hurdle brought new anxiety and fear and dread and uncertainty. *Who's in control here?* I knew it wasn't me.

It was a roller coaster ride, and I was strapped in for dear life. There were times when I was terrified. I could feel my heart speed up and slow down at a moment's notice. *What's happening to me? I feel faint. Am I going to pass out?* I often had internal pep talks with myself. *Pull yourself together and snap out of it. Remember, this too shall pass. This isn't the time to lose yourself.*

Life had indeed become a runaway train, rich with nuance. My journals and notebooks gave me a place to offload some of the heavy, raw emotions. I wrote it all down and let it seep onto the page. Even as I started to misspell words and my handwriting became harder to read, I still captured it all. I emptied it all out on paper. I let it scream and cry on the pages.

The truth is, you're going to feel the way you're going to feel. You have to go through it, because you have no choice. And you don't want anyone sugar-coating it for you. What you feel is real. It's scary and painful, but it's real. Try to deal with it as it comes, then maybe dissect it all later. Analyze it. Put it under a microscope if you need to. Dice it up and put it on a cracker. Do whatever you need to do to process it when you're ready. It's too much to deal with or even try to put into perspective in the moment. You need distance from it. While you're in it, you have no choice but to live it. All of it.

Feeling Scared

Being scared isn't something I talked about very much. I didn't want my fears to manifest by giving them too much air. I wanted to cut off their oxygen supply. But the feeling was real. On occasion, I wrote in my journal about feeling scared, but at home with Kenny, neither of us wanted to go there. We were both in utilitarian mode. *What do we need to do today? What appointments do we have this week? What needs our immediate attention? What do you want for dinner?*

But make no mistake, I was scared out of my mind. Scared of what? Scared of everything. Scared about the cancer spreading. Scared that the chemo wasn't working. Scared about the kind of surgery I was going to need. Scared about the pain. Scared about how I would look if I had to have a double mastectomy. Scared of the cancer coming back. Scared that I might need radiation. Scared of the giant elephant in the room — death. Scared of leaving.

The moment you realize you could die, all you want to do is live. And whether that awareness comes in the form of cancer or something else makes no difference. It is in that moment that you become acutely aware of your own mortality. Death is inevitable. *Momento mori.* That's a Latin phrase that means remember that you must die.

Death is always there, whether we acknowledge it or not. I thought about that a lot when I lost my mom, and that inevitability became even more compounded when I got my diagnosis. But I wasn't ready. I didn't think it was my time and thank God it wasn't. What I do know is it brought me close to the realization of my own impermanence.

So yes, there were days when I was scared *to* death. And others when I was scared *of* death. I think that's only natural, because after all, that's exactly what we are dealing with here — life and death — and death is fucking scary as hell.

Even now, I wonder if I'm a ticking time bomb. And that fear has changed my priorities and my views on life and the people and things I allow in, and those I must keep out.

Bedtime Thoughts

I should be sleeping, but instead, I'm lying in bed, eyes wide open, wondering how I got here. This is what happens when the world grows quiet, and I'm left alone with my thoughts — these racing thoughts. I become my own worst enemy. I allow myself to think the unthinkable and to go places I've tried to barricade off. I force my way through and confront all that stands before me. Warning me to go away.

But I can't help myself. I want to fast forward. I want to know what happens next. I want to know how this ends. They say I'm strong and fierce, yet I'm scared of my own shadow. It feels like a dream, but I can't wake up. *Pinch me. Pinch me. I need to wake up.*

Thoughts are jumping like grasshoppers. I'm thinking about my life. Thinking about my childhood. Thinking about my mom and grandparents. Wondering what they would say to me. Asking them to watch over me. Asking them to work with God to heal me. To save me.

In the quiet of the night, I feel a rare, lone tear making its way down my cheek. I wipe it away and pray — as I do each night — for continued strength. For health. For healing. And for life. Dear God, please give me life.

Anxiety

The voice of anxiety is often much louder than my own. I strain my ears to hear anything else. I have a bad habit. I give anxiety way too much power and freedom. I let him hang out with me all day and deep into the night. I let him lie down next to me when I should be sending him home. I should be firm and tell him I've had enough for one day. But no, thoughts continue to rush around in my head without slowing down. It's hard to keep up with the rhythm of my own breathing. I can hear the pulsating flutters against the walls of my chest. My voice trembles, and my muscles begin to spasm. I compulsively wring my hands.

That's what anxiety feels like for me. And mine isn't purely situational. I've always suffered from generalized anxiety. It often starts first thing in the morning — waking anxiety. I've struggled with it for years. Before my eyes even open, my heart races, and I feel a little faint or nauseous.

For years, my first waking thought was about my kids. *Please let them be OK.* Then that was replaced a few years ago with the stark awareness that my mom was gone. And just like that, it switched again. I would wake up every morning, still in a dreamlike state. And there it was — *oh yeah, I have cancer.* A little jolt to jump-start my day.

It would have been easy to spiral right then and there, but I wouldn't allow myself. I would get out of bed, look cancer right in the eye, acknowledge it, and then walk on past. It became part of my morning ritual. *I have cancer. Ok, got it. Next...* Then I just moved on to the bathroom, brushed my teeth, took a shower, got dressed, ate breakfast, and got on with my day.

And then there was unreasonable anxiety. Yep, that played into the mix too. Whenever Kenny would leave the house to go to his office for the day, I could feel the anxiety rising within me. I recognized it as unreasonable, but it was anxiety just the same. I wasn't even sure what it was about. Mostly, I was just anxious about being alone. I never let Kenny know. He was already working miracles while working a full-time job. I didn't want to add anything else to his plate.

There was also anticipatory anxiety, which has been around me for as long as I can remember. I am unable to stop myself from imagining what and how something will be like before it even happens. Like the night before my first round of chemo. I played the whole thing out in my head. How I thought it would go. Each step. Start to finish. It's a coping mechanism. So, when it's time for the event in question, I can tell myself I already know how it's going to go. *I've been here before, and I'm prepared for this situation. I've already lived it in my head.*

And there's one more form of anxiety that keeps showing up in my life — performance anxiety. This comes from the pressure of having to pretend that everything is normal when doing small things like making phone calls or composing emails.

There was this one day when a client wanted me to sit in on a strategy call. *Strategy call? What the hell? I don't have any strategies. I'm just trying to stay alive and fight my way through this thing, one day at a time. That's all there is. That's all I know.*

Managing Anxiety

Managing anxiety is no easy task, so I've had to figure out what works for me. It's a learned practice. Trial and error. And sometimes, the things that have always worked before are no longer effective. But stress and anxiety are not good when you're battling cancer, so I did what I could to minimize it.

My best in-the-moment strategy was to quickly induce relaxation. A friend taught me this technique twenty years ago. We were on a turbulent flight together on the way to Orlando, Florida. I'm not a great flyer to begin with, so a bumpy flight through a storm was one of my worst nightmares. At one point, I grabbed my friend's arm so hard I'm sure I must have bruised it. This was more than anxiety; this was a full-on panic attack.

I can still hear her voice saying, *Breathe in for a slow count of ten. One ... two ... three ... four ... five ... six ... seven ... eight ... nine ... ten. Now hold your breath for ten. One ... two ... three ... four ... five ...*

six … seven … eight … nine … ten. Now slowly exhale with me as I count. One … two … three … four … five … six … seven … eight … nine … ten.

We repeated that exercise until I was calm. It worked. My breathing returned to normal. Whenever my anxiety feels out of control, I return to my breath. I count to ten.

Here are some of the other things that work for me: having a routine, working out, meditation, quiet time, saying no, removing toxic elements and people from my life, not putting too much pressure on myself, staying in the moment, focusing on a stationary object, not playing the *what if* game, writing, playing the drums, reading, binge-watching TV (comedies, dramas, feel-good shows), getting enough sleep, eating healthy, focusing on the positive, practicing gratitude, understanding and accepting my limitations, accepting help, being around my dogs, and letting things go.

My Reflection

There's nothing like the stark reality of looking in the mirror day after day and night after night and realizing the truth. Gone are my black hair and jagged bangs sweeping over my eyes. My unique edge. My branded locks. My glowing skin and youthful appearance. The sparkle in my eyes. Gone, all gone. Some days I wanted to scream right into that mirror at my own altered reflection. *This can't be right. This is not me. This is not who I am.*

As I stood there glued to this image — my reflection — nothing felt real. It was like looking into a funhouse mirror. I looked strange and distorted. Unrecognizable. My pale, puffy complexion looking back at me. It was my reality staring me in the face. No eyelashes or eyebrows. Not a single hair on my head. I looked small, weak, and fragile. I was sick, and I looked the part.

No matter how long I stared, I struggled to find myself hidden deep within the reflection in the mirror. *I don't feel like myself, and I sure as hell don't look like myself.* I begged. I pleaded. *Make this go away. Let it all be a dream.* But the mirror was unsympathetic to my pleas. I wanted to go back. Way back before any of this. Back to a place where I was still whole. To a place where my mom was still on the other end of the phone. To a place that still made sense to me. But I just stared at myself in disbelief. *How can this be? How can this be me?*

Remembering who you are isn't always easy when you look in the mirror, and you see someone who looks totally different. Almost like you're in disguise. How do you reconcile that? In the end, you have to balance who you are, who you were, and who you are becoming. Everything is different. You are different. You feel different. You look different. But you still have to remember who you are on the inside, no matter how much changes on the outside. You have to keep in touch with yourself. Check in on yourself. Keep looking deeper into the reflection in the mirror, and I promise, eventually you will see it. You will see yourself. And then remind yourself that this is only temporary.

It's Shrinking

By the end of July, after only three rounds of chemo, I noticed I was having a hard time finding the lump in my breast. *Was it my imagination, or wishful thinking, or was it getting smaller?* I wasn't sure, so I let my oncologist tell me at my next appointment.

I noticed she looked a little puzzled while examining me. Then she confirmed it.

"Hmm...Can you still feel your tumor?"

"No, not really. Can you?"

"No, I can't. This is great news because it means your body is responding really well to the chemo, and your tumor is shrinking."

"Oh my God! That's what I thought, but I wasn't sure."

"Yes! Everything is working the way it's supposed to, and you're doing great."

"I can't thank you enough. You are saving my life!"

"Oh, I can't take all the credit. We are doing this together and working as a team, but you're the one doing all the hard work."

"All I can say is that I am so thankful for you and thankful that everything is working."

"Yes, it's a blessing. Your positive attitude has been absolutely amazing. You are like the poster child for how to do chemo."

"Thank you so much! The positivity helps."

She also told me she was going to add an immunotherapy drug to the mix every three weeks, along with chemo. She said this was shown to be beneficial in patients with triple-negative breast cancer. Apparently, it could lead to better response rates and outcomes. Beyond that, I didn't get too hung up on the medical aspects. If she believed this was something that could improve my response rate and outcome, then that's all I needed to hear.

BRCA1 (BReast CAncer gene 1)

As my mom always said, *the plot thickens.*

A few days into August, I tested positive for the BRCA1 gene mutation. Since BRCA1 is often linked to triple-negative breast cancer, I had agreed from the beginning to have a genetic test. I was told this gene mutation leads to abnormal cell growth, which can lead to cancer. So, having this gene mutation significantly increases a person's risk for cancer, namely breast and ovarian. That meant I had an increased risk of developing cancer in my other breast, as well as ovarian cancer. The test confirmed a few things.

First, there was no more wondering whether I would be having a lumpectomy, a mastectomy, or a double mastectomy. I would be having a double mastectomy, followed by the preemptive removal of my ovaries and fallopian tubes. So, one of my earlier questions was answered: *No, I do not get to keep my breasts.*

Secondly, I was told by the genetics counselor that genes and variants are passed from generation to generation. So, this harmful variant could have been passed to me from either of my parents, which meant that Michael could have the gene mutation too. And since I had the mutation, my children had a 50 percent chance of having inherited the mutation from me.

So, Michael and Kendall each agreed to get tested. A few weeks later, they received their results, and they both test positive for the BRCA1 gene mutation. That meant they had the same hereditary predisposition for cancer that I had. This brought an additional level of worry. I was no longer only dealing with my health issues, because my daughter and brother were at high risk too.

CHAPTER 11: LIVING OUTSIDE THE CIRCLE

Sometimes it is after the dust settles that we feel the most alone.

Outside the Circle

People say cancer is lonely and isolating, but it's much more than that. From the moment I was diagnosed, I began living a life that was much different from everyone around me. Their lives were vivid and bold with bright colors, as mine became muted. Normal life stopped. Normal living stopped. It's what I call living outside the circle. Outside of everyone else. By yourself. A party of one. It's like everyone else is on this beautiful island. Palm trees, drinking Piña Coladas, toes in the sand. But all you can do is swim around the outer banks. You keep swimming and swimming, but you are unable to reach them. You must keep a safe distance. Everyone is having fun and living life without you. Your life is on hold, in a state of animated suspension. You are there, but you are not there. It's like living on a different plane from everyone else. Your own dimension. A balloon hovering overhead. Weightless and ungrounded. Floating all alone in this thick atmosphere.

By design, my inner circle is very small to begin with, so to find myself living outside of that tiny sphere was extra lonely and isolating.

But it was also a special place. Almost sacred. People understood it, respected it, and didn't question it. *I'm here, and you're there. No hugging. No touching.* Every encounter outside of my immediate family was at a distance. Outside the circle. That's where sick people dwell.

Girl in a Bubble

Girl in a bubble. That's who I was now. Once I started chemo, my exposure to everyone and everything became extremely limited. And I understood this. It was the sensible thing to do. I felt safer and more comfortable at home anyway. I was immunocompromised, and that became an acceptable excuse for everything.

It was like being in solitary confinement. This voluntary detachment from most everything and everyone. It was both physical and emotional. COVID-19 alarms were still ringing, and no one wanted me to catch it. COVID-19 would have been a complication, and complications were bad.

As time went on, I became increasingly more worried about my exposure to everything. Worried that something might delay my treatment. And it wasn't just about my exposure, but Kenny's too and what he might bring back into our house. It became necessary for him to work almost entirely from home.

I didn't even see Michael that much anymore. Same thing with Kendall and her boys. I was reminded that kids were like little Petri dishes when it came to germs and all the things I needed to avoid. I missed them like crazy, but we settled for lots of phone calls and FaceTime videos.

When my friends came by the house to drop off meals and other goodies, Kenny typically went out to meet them alone while I stayed in the house. But there were times when I really wanted to go out there and say hello, at least from afar. And he let me. It was like being sick from school and having a friend drop by with your homework. You felt like crap and looked like crap, but you still felt well enough to see your friends. Just not well enough to go to school.

The closer I got to my final round of chemo, the more pronounced my worry became. I was worried about anything that could throw a monkey wrench in the process. I didn't want anything to come between me and that final round. That final blow. That last drop of poison that must enter my body. *No delays.*

No setbacks. Just full steam ahead.

I kept reminding myself that it's all about the fight and getting to the other side. Whatever it takes. And I was all in. Yes, at times, it felt like no man's land, but I just kept doing what I was told. Following the rules. When it comes down to it, I am more of a rule follower than breaker. I come from a home with a lot of rules. Growing up, my mom liked to write the rules in calligraphy on parchment paper and post them on the bulletin board in my room and on the kitchen fridge. Not following rules was unacceptable, and I abided.

So, now was not the time to buck the system. I had to focus on the big picture. Do whatever it takes. Live in my protective bubble. My cocoon.

Feeling Fragile

It was like someone had taken a thick Sharpie marker and written all over me: **HANDLE WITH CARE!** *Did I really look so frail and fragile?* When I look back at photos of myself, the answer is a decisive *yes*. The absence of hair, the pale color of my skin, the puffy face, the glassy look in my eyes, the lack of energy, the slow movement, the exhaustion, and the long hours of sleep, all confirmed it. And I felt it too. My own weakness.

When you feel your own physical weakness, it's easy to mistake it for fragility. And maybe it is fragility. *Don't hug me too tight. I might break.* I felt it when Kenny put his arms around me too. His light touch was as if he was afraid to pull me too close. It was strange for me. I've never felt fragile before. I like to think I have a spirit that is unbreakable and the physical strength to match. That's why this feeling was so uncharacteristic. So foreign.

Sometimes I would even feel physically smaller. Like my physical presence had shrunk somehow. It's hard to explain, but it was as if the space I took up in a room or in a chair had dwarfed. There was just less of me. I was a fraction of my former self. This led to some feelings of emotional fragility too, which went hand-in-hand with the feelings of low energy, fatigue, and time spent in bed.

But this was all temporary. Everything was temporary. That's what I kept telling myself. I would get my strength back. I would get my hair back. I would look like myself again. I would be able to do the things I wanted to do. It was all a matter of staying upbeat and believing that the chemo was working, and knowing I would reach the other side. It was the power of positive thinking. That's what got me through many low moments and dark days. *Just weather the storm. You got this.*

Tethered

Before my diagnosis, Kenny and I had plans. Big plans. An exit strategy. To leave Houston and move to Louisiana. My home state. The place where I feel the happiest. The place that connects me to my roots. To my mom and grandparents. To the land, the food, the people, and the culture I love so much. It was calling me home.

On my birthday, just a little over a month before my diagnosis, Kenny and I took a walk through the Japanese Garden in Hermann Park. It's one of my favorite spots in all of Houston. The landscaping is so lush there. You are surrounded by beautiful Japanese maples, dogwoods, crepe myrtles, and cherry trees. There are stone paths, footbridges, and tiny waterfalls. You can hear birds singing, see turtles sunbathing on large stones in the water, and watch as the occasional rabbit hops by. The giant city almost disappears within this secluded Zen-like setting. It's a good place to lose yourself a little too.

That day, Kenny held my hand as we walked through the garden.

"I love this garden, but I hate Houston. When are we going to move to Louisiana?" I asked.

"I don't know. Let's figure out a way to get out of here."

"I'm all for that, but it seems like all we ever do is talk about it. We need a firm plan."

"OK, then I promise this will be the last birthday you have to spend in Houston."

"Really? How are we going to make that work?"

"I'm not sure, but we will figure it out."

"So, next year, on my birthday, my feet are going to be on Louisiana soil?"

"Yep."

"You know I'm going to hold you to that, right?"

"I sure do."

Not only did I spend my next birthday in Houston, but I also spent the one after that here as well. As it happens, I am tethered to Houston, at least for now. It's about my need to stay close to my doctors and the hospital. It's about keeping things consistent. Not rocking the boat. No sudden movements. No uprooting my life. Not just yet anyway.

I was tethered to my home. Tethered to Kenny — my husband, my partner, my rock, my gardener, my service animal. He was my anchor, keeping me from drifting too far before I was ready. During my treatment, I had to lean on him in new ways and trust him to handle everything that needed to happen. To keep things moving in the right direction. To keep track of my meds and manage our food deliveries. To help me find my words and finish my sentences. To keep me present. To take care of me. To reassure me. To pray with me. To love me.

Life Goes On Around You

Sometimes you can't believe it. The world didn't stop. Time didn't stop. Not for you, and not for cancer. Not for a single second. It's all just racing by. Just like normal. And you feel like you're not really a part of anything beyond your disease. Your fight. It's holding you prisoner. Everything is on hold except for this.

Life still goes on all around you. It's a spectator sport, and you're forced to watch from the sidelines. Dates fly off the calendar. Babies are born. People die. Holidays come and go. Birthdays and anniversaries are celebrated. Occasions are marked. People go to work. Friends go on vacation. The seasons change. The time changes. The clock ticks. Time speeds up, and slows down, and moves in all directions.

Meanwhile, your calendar fills up with all your upcoming medical appointments. You have this rigid schedule that wasn't set by you. An agenda that isn't your own. You have your marching orders, and you just do as you are told.

You might feel like you're in a holding pattern, but life doesn't stop just because you have cancer. There is more than just the fear of missing out; there is *actual* missing out.

It's hard sometimes not to feel a little jealous when you look at what other people are doing. I watched a friend document her travels to Italy and Greece through the beautiful photos and videos she posted on Facebook. *I want to go to Italy and Greece. When I get to the other side of this mess, I'm going to see the world.* Much like moving to Louisiana, I haven't seen any of the world now that I'm on the other side of this mess. What's stopping me? I'm not really sure.

Loss of Control

Loss of control. This had become a central theme in my life. That's why I mention it so much in this book.

You realize you're no longer calling the shots in your own life. Sure, you are consulted, but rarely are you given a *real* choice. You are presented with *the* choice, and you're expected to comply. And so, you do. All you want is to beat this thing, so you follow directions and obey your orders.

This makes it harder to see the things you still control. I often had to pause and take stock of what I could still control. I had to keep a mental list. It's a mindset that worked well for me. The two most important things proved to be my positive attitude and my ability to keep moving. Even if I was slower and the intensity was not there, the choice was still mine. *Get up. Get out. Keep moving.*

I also controlled what I shared, what I wore, what I read, what

I ate, who I called, what I watched on TV, what I bought, and, to a certain degree, my own thoughts. Who and what I allowed in, and who and what I pushed out.

In the end, I think it's a willingness to take orders. To trust the process. To remind yourself the only way through is through. And to keep repeating as often as necessary, *God is in control. Trust in Him.*

CHAPTER 12: KEEP MOVING

Cancer can't get you, if cancer can't catch you.

Keep Moving

Keep moving. Those words became my mantra after losing my mom. A reminder that I had to keep going, no matter what. A reminder that it was up to me to carry myself from one day to the next. The words became ingrained in my routine and transformed my lifestyle. *Keep moving.* Those words were like my call to worship. My sacred time to work out. For over two years, my days were driven by my workout routine, not the other way around. It was written in ink all over my calendar. It might as well be written in blood. That's how strongly I felt about it. No excuses. It was my top priority. Commitment, not compromise. Rigid, not flexible.

After my diagnosis, *keep moving* became more of a battle cry for my fight. For staying alive. For beating cancer. I kept telling myself, *cancer can't get you, if cancer can't catch you. So, keep moving!*

Working out, regardless of how fast or slow I was able to move, reminded me of who I was and what I could do. It produced powerful endorphins that lifted my mood while reducing my stress. It allowed me to sweat out the toxins that had been deposited in my body by the chemo. It allowed me to drop some of the emotional baggage that was weighing me down.

Keep moving. I felt the weight of those words every day. They were a constant reminder. The little nudge I often needed. Moving made things better. It made me better. Moving kept my strength up, at least a little. Moving provided a solid connection to my life before cancer. A reminder of the strength I once had. The strength I will have again. *Keep moving. Don't question it. Believe in it.*

Keep moving. Those words reverberated in my head. They were the source of my own resilience. Of what I had already accomplished, and the force that propelled me forward. It was a promise I had made to myself. A firm, unwavering commitment. *Just keep moving. It has served you well, so don't give up on it now. Leverage it. Let it be your guiding principle. The sword for your fight. Your weapon of choice.*

Every day I reminded myself that working out was a gift. *I don't have to, I get to. I control this.* There was such a meditative solace that came with working out, and it gave me some much-needed peace.

Keep moving.

Motivation

Working out is a great motivator. And so, I videoed myself, and I photographed myself, and I talked about what I was doing, how I was doing, and I posted it all on social media. I wanted my friends to see my experience, and what I was willing to do — what I HAD to do — and how I still prioritized my workout routine.

My hope was that my friends would feel compelled to work out with me, because of me, and on some days instead of me. It was a feeling of genuine community and solidarity. I wanted to be a crusader for the merits of exercise, regardless of our circumstances. I wanted to encourage others. I pleaded with them to take my advice. *If I can do this with breast cancer, imagine what you can do. You have no excuse. Get up and keep moving.*

People often said *I was an inspiration*, and whenever I read or heard those words, it would touch me so deeply. I hoped I was indeed inspiring them to do something I believed was vital to their own health and wellbeing.

I never miss an opportunity to remind people how important it is to be self-aware of any changes – big or small – in their bodies. That any change could be a warning sign. That if something doesn't feel right or look right, go see the doctor ASAP. I'm still kicking myself for letting my pain go for as long as I did. Weeks are too long to wait. Days are too long to wait. If

I have any regrets at all, it's that.

Peloton

I could write a whole book about my relationship with my Peloton, and the benefits it has brought into my life since the day it arrived at my door – two years to the day before my breast cancer diagnosis.

The way I see it, my Peloton saved me, not once, but twice. In March of 2019, it had been many years since I had engaged in any real workout routine. Then, I unexpectedly lost my mom. Less than twenty-four hours earlier, I had been researching the Peloton, as I wanted to lose a little weight and get myself into shape. The profound loss of my mom and the complex grief that followed was unbearable. Everything made it worse — eating, drinking, crying — and I could feel myself spiraling. My belief system was crumbling, and I was crumbling along with it. I knew I needed to make some changes.

I don't remember the moment I finally pulled the trigger on the Peloton. I just remember how I felt the first time I rode it. Sluggish and out of shape, yet I forced myself to make it through a twenty-minute beginner class.

Afterwards, I found myself lying on the bedroom floor. Sweat pouring out of every pore. I imagined the sweet release of evil spirits exiting my body. I was exhausted, but aware that something good had just happened. Something monumental. Life changing. It gave the grief somewhere to go. An emotional exit. It was transformative, leaving me spent.

In a way, it was my temporary ticket out. While on my Peloton, I was present. I was able to leave my grief behind for a little while. A brief suspension of all the things I didn't want to think about.

The feeling was addictive, and my Peloton became my gateway drug to other forms of working out — walking, running, lifting weights, yoga, and biking. A switch had been flipped, and I never wanted to turn it off.

It was working. I was toning my body. Eating healthy.

Shedding pounds. Building lean muscle. Increasing my energy and metabolism. There was no stopping me.

For just over two years, my workout routine became increasingly more intense. My Peloton schedule was forty-five minutes, every other day. Then I would lift weights for fifteen minutes, six days a week. And in the afternoons, I would walk for at least hour or more unless it was raining. Running and going for a bike ride sometimes replaced my walks. I had such a good thing going. I looked great, and I felt great.

Then, on the two-year anniversary of my Peloton being delivered, the radiologist delivered the news about my diagnosis. Dates are weird that way. How can two such different events share the same anniversary?

After my diagnosis, I had to accept that my energy level was going to change, and that meant modifying my beloved workout routine. I knew regardless of what changes would be made, one thing was for sure — in whatever capacity I was able, the Peloton would stay in the mix. And my new Peloton goal became: *You don't need to break a record, just break a sweat.*

The nurses in the Infusion Center were encouraging too. They knew all about my love affair with Peloton. A couple of the nurses even had Pelotons of their own. Whenever they asked me how I was doing, I proudly told them I was still riding my Peloton before chemo. They reminded me how incredible that was, considering everything my body was going through.

The way I saw it, my Peloton was the best thing I could do for myself. It didn't matter how fast or slow my cadence was, or how high or low the resistance was, or how many minutes I rode. All that mattered was that I was doing it.

Walking

I had added walking and running to my workout routine during the early days of COVID-19. I was stir-crazy and needed to get out of the house and enjoy the fresh air. It soon became an integral part of my daily routine. Unless it rained, I walked. It gave me a chance to get outside and clear my head. Breathe in some fresh air and enjoy some Vitamin D.

After my cancer diagnosis, I liked to go for a walk as much as possible, but other factors played into the equation.

For one thing, going for walks meant leaving the house. Straying outside of my bubble. And I generally walked alone. Just me, out there in the elements. So, if something happened or if I got too tired to make it back home, that meant I would have to call Kenny or Michael for help. I didn't want to have to do that. So, I made certain that I felt physically able to complete my route before I even stepped one foot outside the front door.

There was this feeling of vulnerability that accompanied me on my walks. I had to be extra careful out there. Stay alert. Be aware of my surroundings.

My walking experience was much different from being on my Peloton. By leaving the house, it gave me a little escape and a feeling of independence. I wasn't cooped up, isolated, and alone. I could wave to neighbors, even though they didn't have a clue who I was. Our neighborhood is strange that way. It didn't matter. I was just happy to be out of the house. To feel the sun on my face. To have a spring in my step and a smile on my face. To record videos with motivational messages.

There was also a remarkable difference in how I looked and sounded in those videos as opposed to the ones I recorded on chemo days. Of all the videos I recorded of myself while undergoing treatment, the walking ones were the best. The best in the sense that I was more relaxed, and in my element, doing something that was normal for me. I sounded more confident, energetic, and cheerful. Just like a little kid on the first day of summer.

Sadly, I didn't get out and walk nearly as much as I would have liked during my treatment. In fact, only fifteen times. How do I know? Because I track my workouts, even when I was going through chemo. The vulnerability issue was mostly to blame for the small number of walks. My family didn't want me walking by myself. They thought it was dangerous, and they were probably right.

Balancing Act

I quickly figured out that it was a balancing act. My need to work out had to be balanced against all the side effects I was experiencing from chemo — namely, the debilitating fatigue. When it hit, it hit hard. All I could do was lie in bed. It was always accompanied by complaints to Kenny because I didn't know how to deal with it. He would stand next to the bed wishing there was something he could do to make it better. To make me better.

There wasn't. I wanted energy. My energy. I had never experienced this level of fatigue, combined with nausea before. I tried to stay ahead of the nausea with my meds, but meds added to that fatigue. Next thing I knew I was asleep. Then awake again. My whole body ached from lying there. My eyes opened and closed involuntarily as I drifted in and out of consciousness. I lost two hours here, three hours there. The TV was on low volume. I needed the white noise. I would much rather have been lacing my shoes and preparing for a walk. Instead, I was fluffing my pillows, tossing and turning, trying to get comfortable.

I was trying to balance my want and need to work out with my low energy level, and my own weakness — real or perceived. And I had no choice but to listen to my body. That meant not pushing myself when I couldn't be pushed.

I didn't want to waste any time or energy on the days when I felt better. I learned to respect the ups and downs and leverage those spikes whenever they happened. It wasn't just a balancing act; it was chemo versus working out. Good versus evil. I had to walk that tightrope.

It was part of figuring out the cycle and working within it instead of against it. Not wasting the days when I felt good enough to work out. Appreciating them as a gift. *It's not a competition. Just do what you can and let that be enough.*

Mind, Body, Spirit

I spend a lot of time lost in meditative thought. Reflective, contemplative thought. The kind that had me racing through my childhood memories, trying to catch the little moments that defined me. Looking back on the things I got right, and the things I got wrong. The people I could rely on, and the ones who let me down. The truths I have been told, and the many lies I would never forgive. The things that made me proud, and the things I have come to regret. The days worth celebrating, and those that have come back to haunt me. Analyzing my relationships, my career choices, and my everyday decisions. It's how I figure out who I really am and what I really want.

After losing my mom, I began the practice of meditation along with my fitness regime. It's a powerful tool for calming the mind and learning to connect with your own breath. To lose yourself by stepping away from all that is heavy. Pushing it aside. All that has been blowing around in your head somehow finds a soft landing at your feet. And, as heavier thoughts come back into focus, you can imagine them floating by on a low-flying cloud. You have the power to let it pass by you or to catch it while it's still in view. The choice is up to you.

Sometimes meditation requires the stillness of both mind and body, while other times, you can achieve peace through movement. At least that has been my experience. Working out provides a natural calming effect for me. It combats my racing thoughts. It shifts my focus.

I remind myself that working out is something I know how to do. *It's my thing.* It keeps me sane, grounded, and balanced. It's my gravity. Restorative and therapeutic. A much-needed break from all that is troubling. A reminder of what I can control and the power of my own strength. It hollows out the anxiety, exposing it for the fraud I imagine it to be. An imposter that has no place here with me.

Health and healing come from that sacred place where mind, body, and spirit collide. The connection is undeniable. All three must be in alignment. All three are needed to make you whole.

Listening to Your Body

One of the most important lessons I learned is remembering how I got here. It was from listening to my body and being aware of changes that didn't feel normal. An undeniable, nagging pain in my right breast that caused me to inspect further. Listening to my body saved my life, and so I trust that.

Listening to your body means a willingness to negotiate and compromise with yourself. To always be attuned and prepared to make changes. Trust me, your body will let you know if today is a workout day. It might even tell you that it's not a workout day at 10 a.m., but change its mind by 3 p.m. It's fickle that way, but trust it. Listen carefully, and you will know when to push and when to back off.

The important thing is the practice of doing, not the length of time or the intensity. It's a routine, a ritual. One that must be followed, even if it must be altered. That's one of the deals I made with myself when it came to running. Physically, I knew I didn't have the stamina to run anymore, so I didn't even try. Walking and riding the Peloton was already a big enough effort. And I was OK with that. It was about modifying, not quitting. *Just keep moving.*

CHAPTER 13: RED WARRIOR

Struggles can be an endless bounty of strength.

New Chemo Cocktail

As I was sitting in the chemo chair about to receive my twelfth round, the clinical pharmacy specialist paid me a visit. He came by on most chemo days to see how I was doing and how well I was tolerating the side effects. He had a soft manner, always smiling even when delivering not-so-great news. And this, was not-so-great news. He reminded me that I would be changing to a different chemo cocktail starting with my next infusion. This new chemo would be what they call A-C (Adriamycin and Cyclophosphamide). Although I knew this change was coming, I hadn't really given it any thought prior to that moment.

"Hi Michelle! How are you doing today?"

"I'm feeling pretty good. The last round really knocked me out though."

"Yes, that is to be expected. So, today is the last day you will be getting Taxol. After today's round, you will have three weeks off to rest and get your numbers up. Then we will begin this next phase of your chemo treatment, which will be kind of an uphill climb."

"Uphill climb? What do you mean?"

"The side effects will become more intensified and compounded with each round."

"In what ways?"

"Namely, nausea and fatigue. They will become more severe and last longer. You might also experience some vomiting, but you will continue to take anti-nausea medication to try and control that. Loss of appetite is also fairly common."

"Great. The fatigue is already so bad, I can't imagine it getting even worse. And nausea and vomiting? No thank you."

"This is a strong chemotherapy drug, and it is very effective, but the side effects can be harsh. You might feel like you can't get out of bed for two or three days, which is perfectly normal."

"Ugh!"

"Yes. That is why these last four rounds will be three weeks apart. We want your body to have a chance to recover between rounds."

He then went over a laundry list of potential side effects. None of them were good. Swollen mouth, mouth sores, diarrhea, shortness of breath, low platelets and white blood cell counts, and a higher risk of infection.

. . .

A few days later, a friend called to see how I was doing. She was one of my breast cancer lifelines. Her journey had taken place a few years before mine, but had been similar — triple-negative, BRCA1, double mastectomy. So, I told her about my new chemo cocktail.

"Oh girl, that's Red Devil. I had that one too."

"Red what?"

"Red Devil. And it's not pretty."

"Seriously? I already know about the side effects, but I haven't heard it called Red Devil. That sounds awful."

"It is, but you will get through it. You've done great so far, so don't let a little thing like Red Devil bother you."

"That's sweet of you to say. You know, I'm just trying my best to fight this thing."

"Well, you are doing everything right. Keep fighting my friend."

"So, why do they call it Red Devil?"

"I think it's because the actual chemo is bright red, and then all the nasty side effects. It looks like blood, which can be hard to look at. I just closed my eyes and slept through most of it."

"Sleeping through chemo tends to work pretty well for me too. I am just nervous about the more intense effects."

"I know, but at least you know what to expect, and that's a big part of it."

"I guess so. I'm just so ready to be done with all of this."

"I hear you, and you will be before you know it. My advice is to take the time to do the things you feel like doing before your next infusion. You will be glad you did, because once you start that Red Devil, you aren't going to feel like doing much at all."

Walk the Walk

My first round of Red Devil was less than two weeks away, and I felt the apprehension growing with each passing day. There had already been so many days when I felt like crap, and I couldn't imagine having that intensify even further. I was nervous just thinking about how my body was going to handle this new chemo. Its reputation had preceded it, and it wasn't pretty. It was starting to get the better of me. I could feel it, especially at night when it was time to go to bed. Kenny saw it too. The uneasiness on my face.

"What's wrong?" he asked.

"I'm not OK. I'm not feeling positive. I'm worried about how I'm going to tolerate this Red Devil chemo. More nausea. More fatigue. Potential for vomiting. All these bad side effects. I don't think I can handle it. I'm already so exhausted, and…"

"Hold on. Try to calm down. You know it isn't good for you to wind yourself up like this. You have come so far already, and you will get through this too. I promise."

"I know, but it just feels like…"

"Take a breath. You know what you need to do, don't you?"

"No. What are you talking about?"

"Tomorrow, you need to go out for a walk, get some fresh air, make a video, and keep that positive momentum going. People count on you to be positive. They count on you to inspire them. They count on you to tell your story. So, trust me. It will make you feel better. It always does."

"I guess so. I haven't walked nearly as much lately as I've wanted to."

"Then, that's what you're going to do. You're on the upswing right now in your chemo cycle, and you have a couple of weeks before you start the Red Devil, so make the most of them."

. . .

It was early October, and the Houston heat had finally begun to cool. It was the perfect weather to go out for a walk, clear my head, and enjoy the brief hiatus. So, that's exactly what I did.

As soon as my feet hit the sidewalk, I felt this renewed sense of freedom. Each step I took was more animated than the last. I was back out there in my natural habitat. Kenny was right. He often was in those days. I needed the fresh air. The wide-open space. The change of scenery.

So, I held my iPhone up, hit the record button, and issued a challenge.

> *Hey y'all! I am out here on this gorgeous day, recommitting myself to walking. In fact, I'm going to be walking every day for the next two weeks. If it's not raining, I will be out here walking. Who's with me? The reason I'm doing this is because I might not be able to do much of anything for a little while. I will be starting the next phase of my chemo, which they say has lots of nasty side effects. The nickname for this chemo is Red Devil, which even sounds scary. So, I'm here walking off my fear, and I'm asking you to do this with me. Every day for two weeks unless it's raining. Commit yourself to walking with me. And after the two weeks, when I'm unable to do it, please do me the added favor of walking for me.*

So, for two weeks, I walked. And, for two weeks, several of my friends indulged me by walking too. There were only three days when I was stopped by the rain. Even then, I would have gladly gotten wet if Kenny had let me.

Red Devil

If anything was ever in need of a rebrand, it was Red Devil. Clearly, A-C had a terrible PR team that needed to be fired. *Red Devil? Really?*

When it was first introduced to me as A-C (Adriamycin and Cyclophosphamide), that didn't sound all that scary. I just figured, chemo was chemo, and that was that. But now, the words *Red Devil* were stuck on a loop in my head.

So, I did the very thing I had banned myself from doing. I Googled it. Just a little. Just enough to confirm what I was already warned about: the harshness of the side effects and potential complications. It was all there in black and white. I could feel the bubble I was already in starting to get even smaller. I would have to limit my exposure to everyone and everything, as my risk of infection was about to increase. And despite all my walking and messages of positivity, I was a tangled mess of nerves.

Luckily, I had an appointment with my oncologist three days before the dreaded first round of this new cocktail. I told her I was feeling apprehensive about what was coming. As always, she was encouraging in her response.

"You don't need to worry about A-C. You are going to do great, just like you have been doing. Your body has responded extremely well to the chemo. I can't even feel the tumor anymore when I examine you, so everything is working and doing what it is supposed to do. Yes, the side effects are a bit more than you're used to, but I think you are going to do very well."

That was all I needed to hear.

Red Warrior

Before I knew it, I was once again settled into my chemo chair in my private little room. Today was the day — Red Devil Day. And I was as ready as I would ever be. *Let's just get this show on the road and check another round off the list. Then let me get home and start my descent.*

Moments later, the nurse walked in.

"So, today's chemo is A-C. I know this has been explained to you, but do you have any questions?"

"No. I just hate that it's called Red Devil. I've been focused on that for the past three weeks, and it kind of freaks me out."

"Well then, I have some good news for you."

"Awesome! I could use some good news."

"A-C is no longer referred to as Red Devil."

"Really? Everyone keeps telling me it's Red Devil."

"Nope. It's now called Red Warrior."

"Seriously? I like that so much better. Thank you!"

"Seriously. And you're welcome."

I didn't know if that was an official nickname or not. It didn't matter. All that mattered was the change that one word had on me. One simple word. It changed my attitude and calmed my nerves. *Warrior.* It's the one word I needed to hear at the exact moment I needed to hear it. I could feel my entire body begin to relax, at least a little bit.

Red Devil needed a rebrand, and it got one. It's funny how changing one word from a negative to a positive can change your whole outlook. It changed the tone for how everything was going to go. *Bring on the Red Warrior.*

Red Poison

My eyes were transfixed on the red liquid that filled the bag that hung from the infusion machine just over my left shoulder. The tube connecting the red poison to my port. I watched in slow motion as the liquid dripped its way into my veins and distributed itself throughout my entire body. The bright red color. You could easily mistake it for blood. Eerie and disturbing. So, I closed my eyes to make it go away. Then opened them again, realizing there was no way to unsee that image. It was burned into my retinas.

I didn't want to remember the optics of that moment, but I

didn't want to forget it either. So, I reached for my iPhone, and for all of ten seconds, I recorded that bizarre vision. The red dripping vision. Not for posting on Facebook, but for me. I just felt compelled to do it. I was entering the lowest point in my treatment. I knew it, and so I captured it.

I was mesmerized by the evil sight. And even though I knew this potent poison would leave me weaker than before, I needed it to deliver the fatal blow to the greater evil living inside me. So, I kept watching it. Living the moment. *Drip…drip…drip.* Until my eyes were too heavy to remain open, and I allowed myself to sleep.

The Decline

The steady, sharp decline came fast. Within forty-eight hours of my first Red Warrior infusion, I could feel myself starting to roll downhill with an intensity I had never experienced before. By the end of the second day, I felt like I was lying at the bottom of a well, unable to pull myself out. I had no strength. No energy. It had all been zapped away, and I didn't have the ability to stay out of bed. I couldn't even stay awake. And I didn't fight it either. I didn't have it in me. No matter how much I hated to admit it, I had to give in.

This was much more than debilitating fatigue. It was like being stuck in a nightmare, unable to wake yourself up. No amount of willing, pleading, or praying made any difference. I had to ride it out. I had to sleep it off. And that's exactly what I did for the next three days. Drifting in and out of consciousness. *Did I even shower?* I must have, but I honestly don't remember how that could have been possible. It took everything in me just to make the short trek from my bed to the bathroom.

My nightstand was the host of all my anti-nausea meds and my stash of Fiji water. I let Kenny keep track of my medication schedule. I didn't trust myself. The stakes were too high. I was afraid I might sleep through a dose or take too much, so I outsourced to my service animal. I felt so bad that I often counted down the hours and minutes until I could take the next dose. The meds made me even sleepier, but the sleep sped up the clock.

I was also suffering through a splitting headache. I could barely lift my head off the pillow. Kenny had to bring food to my bed. He watched as I labored to chew and swallow. Nothing tasted right, and my appetite was gone, along with all my strength and energy. But I needed the fuel, so I forced it down.

There were many days when a microwaved baked potato with a pat butter was all I could stomach. A baked potato was my mom's go-to meal whenever she wasn't feeling well, so there was that. On days when I felt well enough to go downstairs, Max would sit at the table with me while I ate my baked potato. He knows I hate to eat alone. I must have looked pitiful, even to my dog.

I had never felt less like myself. I wasn't sure what feeling like myself even felt like anymore. I was in very unfamiliar territory. I was operating at about 30 percent capacity at best.

And that was the beginning of my new chemo cycle, which would compound with each infusion. Twelve weeks of hell. Twelve weeks of feeling less and less like a warrior.

Struggling

The Red Warrior weeks brought my greatest struggles. Kenny often stood over me while I was lying in the bed groaning. He did his best to reassure me and tell me as many times as I needed to hear it, that I would get through this.

"Look, I know you feel like shit, but just a few more weeks and chemo will be over. But for now, all you can do is take it one day at a time."

"All I can do is sleep and lie here in this bed. I can't stand it anymore. I want to get up, but I have no energy, like none. And I'm so nauseous and my head feels like it's splitting in two. You have no idea how horrible I feel."

"Just let your body rest and recover. No one expects you to do anything except rest right now, so take advantage of that. It's the best thing for you, and you know it."

"But I'm wasting away in this bed."

"No, you're not. You are doing exactly what your body needs you to do. You will get through this, I promise."

Lying in the bed, I could feel myself falling behind. My life was on hold, and I didn't see how it could ever be like it was again. I wasn't sure if I would be able to pick up where I left off, or if I would even want to. No matter how hard I tried, I couldn't visualize what my life would be like once chemo and surgeries and, hopefully, cancer was behind me. *Would it ever be behind me?*

I didn't see a path for going back to where I was. Not exactly, anyway. I've never been one to move backward if I can help it. The only thing that made sense was moving forward from where I was, wherever that might be. That's really all any of us can do. But what did forward look like, this mysterious thing that I hoped would magically transform me?

Time itself moves in strange intervals. I have known it to move forwards and backwards, while at other times standing still. It speeds up, and it slows down, and it takes a pause. Sometimes it feels as if the pause button has gotten stuck, and I am stuck there right along with it. My feet firmly planted in the mud. The sludge. Unable to move. Thankful I wasn't standing in quicksand.

The Bounce Back

I caught on quickly. The rhythm of this new cycle was much different from before. When I was down this time, I went down with a thud, and I had no idea how long it would last. *Three days? Four days? Five days? Who knew?* And the bounce back, when it finally started to happen, was much slower, only offering a slight improvement. That made sense, given the intensity of my decline with each infusion. I had no choice but to be patient and wait it out, even though patience is not my strong suit.

As soon as I would start to feel that bounce, my goal was a simple one: *just stay out of bed.* And I did that again by hiding out in my office whenever physically possible. My handy little life hack. My head heavy as I sat there at my desk. The tingly feeling, like the start of a headache that never manifested. That fuzziness. I was there, but not like I was all the way there. I just wanted time to pass. For the day to pass. And for me to be able to say I got up, got dressed, and did something — anything — besides lie around in bed.

A couple of times, I was able to bounce back enough to cook dinner. My mom used to say, *nothing tastes as good as a home-cooked meal.* She was right. So, whenever I felt good enough to do it, I cooked the foods I craved — the ones that made me happy. Meals like pasta with Bolognese sauce, apricot glazed pork chops with roasted vegetables, Louisiana red beans and rice with andouille sausage. Kenny, though mostly useless in the kitchen, helped me prepare those dinners.

I reminded myself to enjoy the bounce back while it lasted, which was never long enough. It was always overshadowed by the chemo cycle itself, because I knew the bounce back was only temporary. It would soon be erased by the next infusion.

Expect the Unexpected

Always expect the unexpected. It was eight days after my first Red Warrior infusion when it happened. I woke up, got out of bed, and headed towards the bathroom. A few minutes later, I felt like my heart was beating outside of my chest. So, I grabbed my Apple Watch from my nightstand and took my pulse. It read 140 BPM, which is very high considering all I had done was get out of bed.

I sat back down on my bed and monitored my heart rate for the next few minutes. It was still high but coming down slowly. When it got to 110 BPM, I decided to go downstairs and let Kenny know what was happening. By the time I got down the stairs, my heart rate was racing again, and I was audibly winded. I walked into the breakfast room and found Kenny sitting at the table drinking coffee. He watched me as I collapsed into one of the chairs.

"Are you OK? What's going on?"

"No. My heart rate is really high, and I feel lightheaded."

"Oh no! How high?"

"140 BPM when I woke up, then it went down a little, and now it's back up."

"Do you want me to call the doctor?"

"No, not yet. Let's just monitor it for a little while longer. Maybe it will just go back down on its own."

"OK. Maybe some food would help."

"I don't know if I can eat anything right now."

"Sure, you can. Let me make you something to eat, and we'll see if that helps. How about a piece of toast?"

"Maybe..."

"OK, I'm on it."

After a couple of hours, my heart rate returned to normal. Then again, two days later, I woke up to a racing heart. This time Kenny called my oncologist's office and left a message for the nurse. Within minutes, the nurse called back to say that my oncologist wanted me to have an EKG and had referred me to a cardiologist.

While it was suspected that my increased heart rate was caused by chemo, it was better to be safe than sorry.

A few days later, I had an EKG and an appointment with my new cardiologist. Luckily, my EKG was normal, so the cardiologist told me to continue monitoring my heart rate and to use my Apple Watch to detect any signs of atrial fibrillation (AFib). There was one time when it did show signs of AFib, so I sent that readout to the cardiologist.

My erratic heart rate was an issue that persisted throughout my twelve weeks of Red Warrior, but the thing that helped every time was that little suggestion from Kenny: *maybe some food would help.* Whenever it happened, Kenny made me eat something, and it always brought my heart rate down. For a man who can't cook, he makes a mean piece of toast.

The Homestretch

It was there. Right in front of me. I could see it, and I could taste it. The homestretch to the finish line. I could see the flags waving me on. Encouraging me. Supporting me. *You are almost there. You can do it. You're going to make it. Just keep moving.*

It was early December. Only two more rounds of chemo to go. My brain was pretty wacko. I was all over the place. As I look back at my journals, there were so many misspelled words and crossed-out sentences. I hate both of those things. But I was doing good just to be writing in them at all. I knew that, and I embraced it.

I was so sluggish, and I was told my side effects would become even more severe with my last two rounds of chemo. Not what I was hoping to hear, but what can you do? I just took it all in and hoped for the best. Dwelling on it wouldn't have gotten me anywhere, and I definitely had somewhere to go. I had to get to the other side. It was calling my name, and I was ready to cross the line.

So, I did what any fighter would do, I battled with my inner voice. The constant badgering from within. What I wanted to be doing versus what I had to do. There were wild swings between accepting everything that was happening and just doing it. My feelings crisscrossed and overlapped and separated themselves back out again. Like boxers in a ring. You in one corner versus you in the other corner.

Last Round of Chemo

My last round of chemo was on December 30, 2021. It felt important to finish chemo by the end of the year. That way, I could start the new year off fresh, and spend all of January recuperating and preparing for surgery, which would take place in early February. So, naturally, I didn't want anything to get in my way. I was more isolated than ever, and Kenny was too. I wasn't going to let anything come between me and that final round. As the year finished, so would my chemo treatment. It was the perfect, poetic collision.

There I stood, as I had for so many nights, staring at my reflection in the mirror. My naked face and my hairless head. *Tomorrow is the last one,* I told myself. *You can do it. Tomorrow and for the days that follow, you will feel your worst. That's OK. You're ready. You can do it. Just get through this last one. It's your rock bottom, then it's all uphill from there.*

Standing there, facing myself, I felt it all. The full gamut of emotions. Sad, anxious, excited, nervous, scared. Just like the night before my very first round. Ready to get it done. And I looked so unlike myself. A stranger in the mirror. I felt that way too. *Go to sleep, and tomorrow let the red poison do its thing one last time. Let it zap the last drop of your energy. Then ring the bell. Ring it loud. Ring it proud. Let the warm brassy tone vibrate throughout your body. Celebrate the moment. Then go home. Go to the very bottom of the well. Then grab the rope and start to climb out. Step by grueling step. Careful not to go too fast. Careful not to slip. Take your time. Lift yourself up. You can do it. You can fly.*

When the day finally arrived, apart from the big moment of ringing the bell, it was uneventful. That's the way I wanted. I just needed to get through it, get home, and start my final decline.

Ring It Loud! Ring It Proud!

A couple of times during my chemo infusions, I could hear the distinct sound of a distant bell, followed by cheering and clapping. The sounds of joy, relief, and hope. There was no mystery to it. A wonderful warrior had just completed the last round of chemo.

The first time I heard it was early on in my treatment. I remember wondering whether I would want to ring the bell when the time came for me. I thought about all the emotions and drama that get you to that pivotal moment. I thought about the need for celebration. I thought about the linear process of this whole thing. First A, then B, then C. The road would indeed be peppered by each triumph, large and small, and I would want to celebrate. *Yes, I would absolutely ring that bell.*

Now it was my turn. The final round was done, and the Infusion Center team gathered around me as I stood in front of the infamous bell. They were all smiling at me and congratulating me for reaching this incredible milestone.

I was instructed to read the plaque, then ring the bell. So, I handed my iPhone to Kenny so he could video the moment.

The plaque read:

Ring this bell
Three times well
Its toll to clearly say
My treatment's done
This course is run
And I am on my way!

I rang that bell a lot more than three times. Once my fingers wrapped themselves around the cord, there was no stopping me. I was overcome by the sheer emotion of the moment, and everything it represented. I had made it through chemo. I was done. So yes, I rang that bell at least a dozen times.

There was one more ceremonial thing to do. I had to choose a stone. So, one of the nurses presented me with a shallow bowl filled with stones. Each one had a word etched on it. I saw words like *love, laugh, encourage, hope, bravery, friendship*. I dug around in the bowl, hoping to find a stone with the word *inspire* on it, but there wasn't one. Everyone was looking at me, waiting for me to choose my stone. I can't explain why, but I chose the one with the word *laugh* on it. It called out to me, so I took it home. It lives on a bookshelf in my office, along with a couple of healing stones that I brought with me to each round of chemo. They were gifts from Cheryl.

Laugh. It's a good reminder to always laugh. No matter what life throws at you, find the humor.

CHAPTER 14: KEEPING THE FAITH

God has put me where I need to be when I need to be there. And I believe that with all my heart.

Faith in God

When I was a kid, I used to say my prayers every night before I went to sleep. I don't know what happened to that practice or why it stopped. It just kind of fell off somewhere, probably when I was a teenager. But there are moments in our lives when we need God's attention. So, we turn to our faith. We turn to prayer. And we turn to God.

After my mom's death, I found myself in need of a little help in the spiritual department. There is no doubt that Joanne was sent to me by my mom and God. They clearly worked together on that one. As I've said before, Joanne is many things to me, including my spiritual guide.

During my treatment, we spoke on the phone every day. And on my roughest days, her voice had an immediate calming effect. As soon as she said, *hello sweetheart,* suddenly everything was a little better.

I took comfort in her words, especially whenever she recited verses from the Book of Psalms (*Tehillim,* as it is known in Hebrew). It helped me find a little peace and healing in the midst of my turmoil. Lord knows I was struggling to find my footing on the strange path that was thrown in front of me. So, I listened intently to the heartfelt tone she used when expressing the words that she holds so dear.

Joanne often reminded me to lean on my faith and trust in God. She would say, *God knows all things — past, present, and future. He knows our thoughts, and he knows our hearts, and he knows our needs. So, we must put our trust in Him. Let go and leave it with God.*

Those words gave me hope. The notion that God was in

control somehow lessoned my burden and helped guard against unwanted fear.

Many times since my diagnosis, I found myself pouring over books about Judaism and reading from sacred texts. Looking for meaning, hope, and healing. Looking to God. Sometimes I even wrote down a passage or two. *The Tehillim* was a book I dipped into the most. It was always next to me on the left side of my desk.

Rarely in my life had I picked up *The Holy Scriptures* and read from it, but I did that too. I kept my mom's copy within easy reach. The gold leaf pages are stuffed with the four-leafed clovers she collected as a child. The pages are old and crinkly, and the font is almost microscopic, but it's the one I reach for over and over again.

In times of crisis, I tend to cling to my faith. And though there have been many times when I've felt that my prayers have gone unanswered, my faith remains unwavering. My relationship with God is a simple one — it just is. I walk blindly, though never alone because God is always with me. Not knowing what lies ahead, and taking the next step anyway, is the very essence of faith. It carries me through those blind spots.

So, I returned to the bedtime prayers of my youth. Each night I would lean over and turn off the lamp that sits on my nightstand. It's the same lamp that sat on my mom's nightstand. The same one she would reach over and turn off each night. I would quietly lie there on my back, beneath the soft glow of the light reflecting from my window. My gaze would become transfixed on the ceiling fan above me. Then, I would take a deep breath, close my eyes, and speak from the depths of my heart. Praying to God. Asking for the simple gift of life. *My life.*

Faith in Others

It's more than faith in God, it's also faith in others. Faith in your family and friends. Faith in your medical team. You are trusting them with your life. To get you through this, whatever it takes.

To be there *with* you and *for* you. To lift you when you are unable to lift yourself. To inspire you. To encourage you. To support you. To feed you. To be your service animal. To be strong when you are weak. To believe that everything they are doing is for you and to heal you. To save you. Because they love you.

So, while I was leaning on my own faith, I appreciated that others were leaning on theirs too. When you are ill and fighting for your life, every prayer counts. It's not the time to question to whose God one prays. It's about believing in the power of prayer and allowing it to comfort you. And to feel it – I mean really feel it – in every fiber of your being.

I wasn't shy about asking for prayers. And my family and friends were very generous in answering the call. So many people told me they were praying for me every day. They wrote it in the comments on my Facebook posts and in text messages. They told me on the phone. They sent me cards and notes. They emailed me. They made sure I knew. I can't explain it, but I know in my heart that it made a huge difference. Yes, you have to keep the faith, but it's equally important to let others keep it with you and for you.

Faith in Yourself

Faith in yourself is about believing that you can and will get through this — whatever *this* is. There will be moments of fear and doubt and anguish, but they must be overshadowed by your own strength and unbridled will.

For me, there was only one outcome, and that was to be cancer-free. I never thought about or imagined any other possibility. Sure, there were moments when I was scared that I might not get through this, and that I might die, but I knew I had to pull myself back as quickly as possible. Fleeting thoughts were OK, but I wouldn't allow them to detract from the mission at hand. I never stopped believing I would get through this. And I didn't allow negative thoughts or negative people to permeate that belief in any way. I did whatever it took to distance myself from all things negative.

Even now, if I start thinking too deeply or look too closely at what happened, everything might seem like it was a bit of a mess. But it was not a mess. Not everything, at least. That's something cancer has taught me. Strength prevails. Even in my weakest moment, I persevered, because I had too. Everything followed a methodical process that took me from A to Z. From diagnosis to healing. But I knew there was always that danger of allowing my thoughts to sink too low. To think too far ahead about the future and what could happen. And there are just certain places I never want to visit, not even in my head.

One of the things that helps me, is practicing the art of positive visualization. There is almost a meditative quality to this practice, which is simple to do. You just visualize a positive situation for yourself. It takes you outside of your current situation and lets you focus on how you want to feel and see yourself and your life in the future. It provides a positive vision to accompany positive thinking.

During the lowest points in my battle, positive visualization helped me to see myself on the other side of this illness. Sometimes I would close my eyes, and other times I would just gaze into the mirror until I could see it. That vision of myself – healthy and cancer-free, with a full head of hair, eyebrows, eyelashes, and looking fit. A giant smile on my face, ready to take on anything and everything that came my way.

Chai/18/Life

I'm pretty sure I have obsessive compulsive disorder. It's self-diagnosed, but nonetheless real to me. One of the ways it manifests itself is through my compulsive need to count. I count everything. Each step as I climb a flight of stairs. The number of times I stir my coffee. The number of tiles on a ceiling.

My magic number has always been eighteen. That's not the same as a lucky number. That's much different. To me, the magic number is the one I want to reach when I am counting something. For example, as I climb the stairs, I am thinking, *just let me reach eighteen before anything happens. Before the phone rings, or the dog barks, or I hear Kenny's voice.* I have no idea why I do this; it's a compulsion.

Why eighteen? In Judaism, eighteen holds great significance, because it symbolizes *Chai,* which means *life.* In the Hebrew alphabet, each letter has a numerical value. The word Chai is spelled using the Hebrew letters Yud (ten) and Het (eight). Together they make eighteen. So, Chai is eighteen, and eighteen is life.

It's the number I often see when I close my eyes. It sometimes flashes like a neon sign, making sure I see it. It's synonymous with life — my life. *Think about eighteen. Meditate on eighteen. Stir my tea eighteen times. Just let me reach eighteen.*

And then I ask God, *please let there be life. Continued life. Chai.*

. . .

There is this fragility to life. I learned that the night I lost my mom. It causes us to appreciate each other a little more and hold on a little tighter. Later is not guaranteed. I try not to think about it, but it's always there, twirling around my head like a prima ballerina. It's about how quickly things can change and have the power to break us when we least expect it. And what we can do to fight back. It's when physical strength fails us, and we are forced to rely on our internal strength. And yes, the strength of God. We must blindly trust in that and trust in Him. Even when we are angry at God for what has befallen us or someone we love. Especially then. Strength through faith. Strength because of faith. An unbreakable bond that will be tested over and over again.

High Holidays

Kenny and I sat side by side in our matching navy recliners in the living room. It was *Erev Rosh Hashanah* (Rosh Hashanah Eve). We had decided to live-stream the service from the synagogue. This was nothing new; we had been live-streaming services for a few years now. So, that felt completely normal.

What was extraordinary, was my unexpected, renewed connection to every prayer. My heart hung onto every word the rabbi spoke in Hebrew and in English, as tears streaked my cheeks. I felt it all. The words. The meaning. The absence of those who once loved me the hardest. My stunning Maw-Maw Pearl, who always sat next to me in temple when I was a child. I could still see her beautiful long legs and Stuart Weitzman heels. Holding my hand and smiling down at me as I twisted her emerald ring around her finger. I could still feel her hand giving mine a little squeeze.

Heads turned whenever she entered the room. Her white hair and sky-blue eyes made it impossible to look away. She embodied elegance, style, and class.

And then there was my mom, who was still meant to be here. Equally as beautiful as my Maw-Maw Pearl, but with an elegance, poise, and grace all her own. Heads turned for her too. Oh, how I wished they would both materialize, if only for a minute, to hold my hand and tell me everything was going to be OK.

The Book of Life

On Rosh Hashanah it is written, and on Yom Kippur it is sealed.

In Judaism, the Days of Awe are the ten days that begin on Rosh Hashanah and end at the close of Yom Kippur. It is a time of deep introspection, as we seek forgiveness from God for all our misdeeds, as well as forgiveness from those we may have wronged during the previous year. It is believed that on Rosh Hashanah our fate is decided, and on Yom Kippur it is sealed. Who will live, and who will die.

We ask God to *inscribe us in the Book of Life*. I had spoken those words in unison with my family, along with other members of the congregation, for as long as I could remember. I had observed this deeply solemn time and its traditions my whole life. I had recited the prayers. Some in Hebrew, some in English, some in both. They were ingrained in my soul.

But this time, each word of each prayer hit a little differently. The words were not just rolling off my tongue; they were flowing like a river from my head to my toes. I felt the intense reverberation of each syllable. I heard the familiar cracking of my own voice as I spoke. Connecting like never before. Embracing my faith like never before. Honoring my personal covenant with God and understanding the significance like never before. Praying for forgiveness. Praying for life. I needed God to hear me like never before. To hear my plea, and to inscribe me in the Book of Life.

Peace/Shalom

I have been searching for peace since the day I lost my mom. *Peace (Shalom* in Hebrew) was the word I assigned to myself as a goal for the year 2021. Instead, my word that year became *cancer.*

How do I reconcile these two words with completely opposing views? How can I have peace and cancer? Is it possible for the two to coexist? *Not really.* It was either one or the other, and I didn't have a choice in the matter. So, my word for 2021 would demonstrably be *cancer.*

But that didn't mean I stopped looking for peace, or that I put it on hold. Instead, I continued to ask God to grant me peace — peace through health and healing. And I kept all manner of things that didn't aid in my health and healing as far away as possible. That meant making some difficult decisions about who and what would have access to my life.

I've mentioned that so many times in this book because it's some of the best advice I can give. When you find yourself in a situation where you control so little, you can rope yourself off from those who aren't really cheering you on. From those who would do you more harm than good. They're not worth the headspace. Instead, focus on the fight and what you must do.

What you need to do. Leave everything else untouched as if it doesn't even exist. Trust in yourself, and trust in God.

. . .

Over the last couple of years, I've thought a lot about the Serenity Prayer, and how it relates to me and my cancer journey. Before my diagnosis, I was familiar with the prayer, but I had never really taken the time to ruminate on the words or study the meaning.

> *God, grant me the serenity to accept the things I cannot change,*
> *The courage to change the things I can,*
> *And the wisdom to know the difference.*

Early into my diagnosis, a friend of mine sent me the Serenity Prayer in a text message. I remember sitting there holding my phone, reading the words repeatedly. Letting them sink in. *Serenity…accept…courage…change…wisdom.*

So, I asked God to grant me the serenity to accept my situation, my diagnosis, the side effects — all of it. Those were things I couldn't change, no matter how hard I tried. So instead, I looked for the things I could change and control, and I focused on those. I accepted my plight, my reality, my diagnosis. I had to. I knew I couldn't waste precious time worrying about the things I couldn't control. I didn't have to like it, but I did have to accept it. It was more of an acknowledgment of what was and what must be. And even if I couldn't control the events as they unfolded, I could at least control how I acted and reacted to them.

This understanding is at the very root of acceptance. You must give in to it, because with acceptance comes peace. And peace follows every storm.

Blessings & Gratitude

I believe that a life filled with gratitude is a life well-lived. So, why is it often so easy to forget to count our blessings? I think we are all guilty of that one. But we need to remember that gratitude is the most important ingredient for a healthy attitude. When it's missing, the whole recipe turns to shit.

Even during the throes of treatment and debilitating fatigue, I made it a point to never stop giving thanks. Thanks to God, and thanks to the many people who picked up their swords and fought along with me every day through their prayers, healing thoughts, and encouraging messages. Even those who hardly knew me or didn't know me at all.

One day a friend of Michael's showed up at my door with a pot of Gumbo and a huge container of potato salad. *Who does that? Who makes food for someone they don't even know?* The kindness and generosity blew my mind. It made me want to be a better person. To put the needs of others before my own. To stand in the kitchen all day and cook for a stranger.

It's an important lesson. And I will never stop saying *thank you.* And I will never stop trying to pay it back and pay it forward. To appreciate and show gratitude for all the love, support, friendship, encouragement, prayers, and good vibes that were sent my way.

In Hebrew, the term *Hakarat HaTov* means recognizing the good. It means *gratitude.* So, for me, yes, I had cancer, but I was also grateful for the love of my husband and family and the many people who gave of themselves during my time of need.

It's a reminder that no matter how dark it gets, there is always light. And, in the midst of darkness, we often find the brightest stars. Sometimes you look for them, and sometimes they just appear.

Someone Is Watching Over You *

My mom. My North Star. She is gone. Suddenly and shockingly obliterated from my sky without warning. How will I ever find my way in the darkness?

Faith. It leads me blindly out of the darkness and helps me find my way. Steadying my feet on uneven land. Allowing me to stand up again after a traumatic fall. Regaining my balance and watching as the path forward reappears from dust. It is newly paved just for me. It is my path. An altered path. An unexpected journey I never thought I'd take. And there is light. Flickering in the distance. Summoning my next step. So, I tell myself, *just go*.

. . .

Someone is watching over you *. I stare at those words several times a day. They are posted on a small marquee board that sits on my kitchen counter. The letters deliberately placed by my mom's own hand. I wonder what compelled her to use that small board to write her message. The most personal gift to me from my non-writer mother. I am mesmerized by those words. Eternal and deeply transcendent.

Someone is watching over you *. My mom's final message to me. The words now permanently etched into my skin. A tattoo that I share with Kendall. She indulged me for my birthday and agreed to get matching tattoos. The words of my mother memorialized on the inside of my left forearm. A constant reminder that she is watching over me. That she will always be with me. That she never left. My North Star is visible anytime I need to see it. And the words of my mom let me know she will always be there. Always watching over me.

My mom would absolutely hate that I got a tattoo. She wouldn't understand it any more than I understood Kendall tattooing my name on her arm many years ago. My mom wouldn't understand why this tattoo was so important to me. She would probably tell me I had mutilated my body and remind me that a tattoo is forever. *Yes, Mom. That's the point.*

Not everything that is meaningful to you is meant to be understood or approved by anyone else. Permission comes from within.

Monarch Butterfly

A fortuneteller once told me that my Maw-Maw Pearl appears to me as a Monarch butterfly. Elegant, graceful, and majestic with a delicate sprinkling of magic.

A couple of weeks after my final round of chemo, I walked outside of my house just in time to catch a glimpse of a beautiful Monarch butterfly, fluttering its wings on my pebble driveway. A rare and captivating sight. The slow movement of the wings reminded me of Maw-Maw's long eyelashes, blinking in unison to reveal her gorgeous blue eyes. I've never known anyone else who possessed such a regal beauty. It earned her the nickname of *The Princess*. And she was truly *my* Princess. The most special person you could ever meet. You could feel it when she walked into a room. Even the walls changed.

Whenever I am lucky enough to see a Monarch butterfly, it tells me that my grandmother is close by. Visiting me from above. My guardian angel, here to protect me and give me hope. It reminds me of the symbolism often attributed to butterflies — change, transformation, hope, renewal, spiritual growth, new beginnings. And, despite its delicate appearance, the Monarch butterfly is said to represent strength and endurance.

That's how I still see my grandmother, the embodiment of strength and endurance. One of God's most beautiful creatures, with a love that refuses to die.

That butterfly was my grandmother's way of telling me that although I might feel more like a caterpillar, I would soon be a butterfly. Change, transformation, hope, renewal, spiritual growth, and new beginnings were all coming my way.

CHAPTER 15: CHECKING IN WITH MYSELF

Fear not the glass half empty. Tomorrow is on its way.

Catching My Breath

There were thirty-five days between my last round of chemo and my *big surgery,* as I like to call it. From a medical standpoint, it was a time for me to get my blood cell counts up in preparation for surgery. But for me, it was also a moment to take a breath and take stock. A lot had happened already, and there was still more to go.

I was wiped out from chemo. As promised, the side effects were extremely severe, so my last round was my worst round. There was a longer period of draining decline, followed by a slow and steady climb back up. And as I began experiencing the bounce back, my mind started doing its thing. *Hello stress, anxiety, nerves, fear. Welcome back!*

Yep, the weeks leading up to my big surgery were fraught with anxiety. My nerves had reached a tipping point. I was cruising into the most pivotal part of the process — surgery and what the pathology report would reveal. So, I took this time to assess where I was, everything I had been through, and look ahead to my impending double mastectomy. *Bye-bye boobs.* I was standing at the intersection of drama and trauma. It's no coincidence that those words sound so similar.

I was mourning the loss of my hair, my eyelashes, my eyebrows, my creativity, my freedom, my self-confidence — all the while preparing for life-altering, body-changing surgery. My breasts were no longer mine. They were trained assassins. They were diseased and had to go. They were being surgically removed. I understood that, and I accepted it, but the thought of it never

155

got easier. I had already given up so much, and now they were going to take two of my favorite things. *Oh well. It is what it is.*

I Don't Look Like Myself

Every time I turned around, there it was again. That distorted reflection in the mirror. Throughout the last several months, my appearance had grown progressively worse. *Who is that stranger in the mirror? That can't be me.* Oh, but it was me. An odd, altered version. I never got used to it. Never! That pitiful image glaring back at me. The small amount of peach fuzz on my head holding on for dear life. The missing eyelashes and brows. The puffy cheeks and pale complexion. The watery eyes. The petrified look underneath it all.

More than anything else, it was about the hair. That was the hardest thing to see. There were several times when Kenny talked about shaving his head. Partially as an act of love, and partially because he had been threatening to do so for years. Each time I said *no.* Each time I told him he had to have the hair for both of us right now. *Shaving his head? DENIED!* Having the hair for both of us was a serious honor, not to be taken lightly.

Many nights he would lean over me in the bed, and I would whisper, "Let me touch your beautiful hair. It's so full and soft. You now have the hair for both of us."

"Yeah, my hair is really beautiful, ha-ha."

"No, seriously, let me touch it again. Lean back over."

And he would indulge me again and again. That was a little routine we had going. Our new form of intimacy.

Routines make things seem normal. That's why I kept up the routine (or charade) of getting up in the morning and following all my usual steps. Taking a shower and washing the few strands of hair left on my head. Putting on my makeup, my lipstick, my perfume, my jewelry, and my clothes. Standing in my closet, choosing the baseball cap *du jour.*

Then doing the whole thing in reverse each night. Removing all those things that made me look and feel as close to normal as possible. My mom's voice bookending the whole thing. *If you look better on the outside, you will feel better on the inside. Accentuate the positive. Don't forget to exfoliate. And moisturize, moisturize, moisturize.*

Surreal

Surreal. It's a word people use so casually. But, when you experience it for yourself in such a profound way, you finally understand the meaning.

Sometimes it felt like I was looking at myself through a window instead of a mirror. I was certain I must be outside looking in, observing myself from afar. No way was that my reflection. I must be watching TV or a movie. Maybe it was a dream. Maybe I imagined the whole thing. And then I'd snap myself out of it. Telling myself to just get through these next few weeks, and the surgery, and the healing, and the recovery, and then, just maybe, life would begin to snap back into place.

I thought if I stared at my head long enough, I could wish my hair into existence. Now that chemo was over, it was free to grow. But it was no use — no change, no hair, not yet. *When will it start to grow back? Will it be all grey, curly, and coarse to the touch?* I tried to imagine.

Then I picked up my iPhone and looked at photos from only a year ago. The straight black shoulder-length hair with my own brand of edginess. My fit body. My makeup — mascara and real eyebrows. My skin — smooth and even-toned. The genuine smile on my face. Knowing beneath that smile was my confidence and belief that things were getting better. That I was getting better.

I had made big, positive changes in my life just before getting cancer. And I was trying to find some peace. I could almost see it in the distance, but it was a little out of focus and still just out of reach. And now I knew the reason why. There was this other storm brewing, just beneath the surface of my right breast. No one forecasted it. This was a surprise storm.

And now, as I faced the mirror, my own face unrecognizable, I knew I had to keep climbing while digging deep down inside. I wasn't sure if I would ever look like my old self again. Someone different was getting ready to emerge, but I had no clue who that would be.

I Don't Feel Like Myself

Not only did I not look like myself, but I didn't feel like myself either. I'm not sure which one was worse. Separately they were awful, but combined, they were unbearable. I was detached from my hair, my boobs, and the person I was before cancer. That exercising maniac who was drowning her grief in sweat.

My train of thought was unfocused, and every time I opened my mouth to speak, I could feel my confidence slipping a little more. *Was there an imposter in my body, or was I the imposter in someone else's?* It was hard to tell. You just know when you don't feel like yourself. I had undergone six months of chemo, which had taken so much out of me.

Routines helped in the moment, but the day-to-day was increasingly difficult. Much more so than I ever confessed. That was because I didn't want to further burden those around me. I didn't want them to worry about how I was feeling emotionally on top of everything I was experiencing physically. This added to my feelings of isolation and loneliness. It was true that much of what I was feeling was tied to the side effects of chemo. So, I reminded myself that these feelings — like everything else — were only temporary.

With each passing day, I was moving further and further away from my last round of chemo, and those side effects were slowly dissipating. I just had to be patient and give it time.

Still Moving

I believe in keeping promises, especially those I make to myself. So, I was determined to keep the most important promise of all — *keep moving*. And I had. Up until the last few days before my big surgery, I continued to ride my Peloton and take a few walks.

I was still lifting weights a little too. I had kept to a routine. And I was ready for surgery. The month in between my last chemo and surgery allowed for a nice bounce back, and I was taking full advantage of it.

My Peloton had been that one constant. That relic from my old life, my old routine, my old body, and the old me. I had to keep riding. I had to keep moving.

And then it happened. Just eight days before my big surgery, I hit a huge milestone — my 600th Peloton ride. To be able to reach that goal before my surgery was critical for me, so I did everything I could to make it happen. It was symbolic. It was an achievement. It was proof that I still had it in me. *Yes, I can still do this, even with cancer.*

Self-Indulgence

As a means of trying to balance or *reward* myself for all the losses associated with cancer, I was a frequent participant in self-indulgence. *Eat the cookie, have more cake, order a Muffuletta from New Orleans, splurge on a new fountain pen, order more books, buy a new pair of comfy shoes, upgrade my iPhone.* The way I saw it, I deserved a few creature comforts to balance out the many discomforts. So, I didn't hold back. I indulged.

Cake was a big one, because hello? It's cake. And luckily, I enjoy baking almost as much as I enjoy cooking. It's cathartic, and it's one of the ways I soothe myself. *Calories? Who cares!* Cake is what I allowed myself. It sure didn't replace hair, but it was the only trade I could make. It was like *cancer took my hair, so I'm having cake. Try to stop me!*

Having cancer is a good excuse for just about anything. Gaining or losing a few pounds, taking a nap, being forgetful, not working, looking like crap, needing help – you name it. No one is going to tell you *no* if they can help it. They want to see you having these isolated moments of pleasure. It shouldn't be *all cancer all the time.* You need breaks. And smiles. And laughter. And self-indulgence. And most definitely, cake.

Conversations with Mom

We never quite recognize the moment before everything comes crashing down and falls apart. It always takes us by surprise. When I went to bed the night before my mom died, there was this feeling of dread mixed with anxiety. I remember it so well. I knew something wasn't right, but I had no idea what it was. The whole world seemed a bit off, like it was teetering on its axis.

I had that same feeling just before my diagnosis. I didn't recognize that moment either, I just knew something was off. But breast cancer was the last thing on my mind.

By all accounts, I was healthy. So, I never saw it coming. And I had to face the whole thing without my mom. Without talking to her on the phone several times a day. Without her coming with me to chemo. Without her rubbing my feet. Her absence was ever-present. That giant hole in my heart that will never refill. As she would have said, *you picked a fine time to leave me, Lucille.* Yep, she sure did.

Did cancer pull me out of my grief? In some ways, yes. In other ways, no. Grief is always there; it just evolves. And cancer demanded my full attention. So, without thinking, I just shifted gears.

So, my grief took on a different shape and form, lingering in the background. It took on a different meaning and manifested itself in a new way. I like to call it: *conversations with Mom.*

Her death was so shocking and sudden, that we still had a lot of unfinished conversations. Many unanswered questions. Zero closure.

Since her death, I talk to her every day. There's kind of this blurry line between talking to my mom and talking to God. Mostly those conversations take place in my head and in my heart, but when I feel like I really need to be heard, I speak out loud. Sometimes I even shout. There is so much I need to tell her and share.

When she was alive, we often had late-night texts and calls that lasted for hours. No doubt, she would have plenty to say about me having cancer. I tried so hard to imagine her words and how she might comfort me. I think she would have been freaked out and frightened, and it might have been me who ended up comforting her. Keeping her optimistic and reassuring her that I would get through this and be OK.

This was uncharted territory. Neither of her children had ever been this sick before. She was a chronic worrier, and she passed that worry down to me and Michael. Perhaps she also had the BRCA1 gene mutation and passed that down to us too. We will never know.

Would I have told her about the lump in my right breast? *Yes.* And she would have asked me if I wanted her to go with me to the doctor. Chances are, I would have said *yes.* But what would she have said when I was diagnosed? That's where I come up short. Though she was rarely at a loss for words, I don't think she would have had words for this. She would have reinforced the notion that we don't have breast cancer in our family.

Not only did I wonder what she would say to me, but I wondered how she would look at me too. It would have been hard for her to look at me and see how fragile I looked. There is a part of me that's glad she never had to see me like that. And that I never had to see that look on her face — the one she wouldn't have been able to hide.

I also know she would have hated me going public with my diagnosis and treatment. She didn't really understand the point of social media. She wouldn't have understood the videos from the chemo chair or my candor about everything that was happening. She wouldn't have been able to relate to looking and feeling terrible and putting myself out there anyway.

Still, every morning when I wake up, her face is often the first one I see. I have a photo that sits just a short distance from my bed. Sometimes as my eyes begin to open and pull me away from my dreams, I see her and say, *good morning, Mom.* Other times I look at her picture and say, *can you believe this shit?* Or *please tell me I'm going to be OK.* Or, *did this come from you?* Her eyes follow my every movement throughout my room, just the same as they did in life.

There are lots of nighttime visits too. Dreams so vivid they must be real. Her body so close she had to be there. That crusty-eyed feeling when I wake up that tells me the tears weren't only in my dreams. That pain in my heart and sick feeling in my gut that says it really happened. That eerie warmth is all too familiar.

I often listen for those creaks that happen in the night. Furniture popping and little noises that seem to come from the house itself. But it's much more spiritual than that. It wakes me up. I often imagine it's the sound of my mom's footsteps pacing the floor around me. Letting me know she's with me. Telling me everything is going to be OK. That I'm going to be OK.

She couldn't sleep, just like me. Her racing thoughts and constant worry caused her to roam the halls. And now, perhaps, she roams mine too.

Mustache

Hormone replacement therapy. That was the last in-person conversation I had with my mom, just four days before her death. We were at family dinner, and I was feeling fat and bloated and menopausal. Something was telling me it was time to stop taking estrogen, which had been prescribed for me as a hormone replacement therapy. I had been taking it for a few years, and I was certain it was responsible for making me feel like crap. Maybe it was, maybe it wasn't.

"Do you want a mustache?" Mom asked.

"No, but I don't feel very good taking it anymore, so I want to talk to the doctor about maybe lowering the dosage or just going off of it completely."

"Mustache!"

"No. I just want to talk to him about an alternative."

"Suit yourself, but don't come crying to me when you have a mustache."

"If I grow a mustache, I will just wax it off."

"To be continued…"

. . .

That night ended with two familiar things: fortune cookies, and a call later that night with my mom. She loved fortune cookies, and she saved the fortunes. All of them. Hundreds of them over the years. She would often text me a picture of her fortune on nights when we were apart. Her texts always read, *And the fortune cookie says...*

Mom saved the fortunes, and I saved the texts. This was one of my favorites: *And the fortune cookie says...Even the toughest of days have bright spots. Just do your best.* Sometimes a message from above shows up in a fortune cookie.

Silver Linings

So, how do you stay positive? People asked me that all the time. Sometimes it was hard. My strategy was to look for silver linings. No matter how small, I knew they were always there.

Having cancer was awful, but that doesn't mean everything that happened because of it was awful too. It was also punctuated by lots of laughter, surprises, and an outpouring of love, support, and friendship. So, it wasn't all bad or sad all the time. There were many silver linings.

For one thing, Kenny and I were given the gift of spending more time together. It might not have been for the reasons we would have hoped, but it was quality time just the same. And for the most part, I could spend my time however I wanted and needed to, without too much pressure from the outside world.

I was also given the luxury of a lower-maintenance lifestyle. I could be showered, dressed, and ready to go in under thirty minutes. No hair to dry or style, and nothing to shave. Not to mention the cost savings. No over-purchasing of hair products. No need for hair color.

Some days the only decision I had to make was which baseball cap to wear. I had old ones, new ones, and gifted ones. Mostly I went for the baseball caps because they were soft, comfortable, and easy to wash. Towards the end, I started reaching for the same one every day. A black Adidas baseball cap Kendall had given me.

The weather no longer bothered me either. When it rained, it rained. It no longer mattered how high the humidity was outside. There was no hairstyle to mess up. None whatsoever. I could just step outside without caring about that first hair-wilting inhale of thick air. And we are talking about air so thick you could smell it — wet and moldy with a tinge of nasty.

Even the heat of the hot Texas summer didn't make me flinch. None of the small things seemed to matter anymore. They had all fallen away. And it was liberating.

It's about finding the positives amid a traumatic experience. It shows you what you're made of — it tests you and redefines you. It gives you the space to become more connected to yourself and to those who matter. It allows you to come to grips with your own strengths and weaknesses. You learn to live with dependence over independence. And you learn to let go of all the crap that doesn't matter anymore. You remove inhibitions. You embrace your own vulnerability. You look at your life and learn to be OK with all the cracks, glue, and tape. Accepting and appreciating the imperfections.

CHAPTER 16: MAKE MINE A DOUBLE

The sun sets on today, whether we are ready to see it go.

Hurdles

There were several hurdles to clear before surgery. I had appointments with my cardiologist, my breast surgeon, my reconstruction surgeon, my oncologist, my endocrinologist, and my OBGYN. I also had a CT scan, an echocardiogram, and an immunotherapy infusion. Somehow, I even managed to slip in a manicure, just a couple of days before surgery.

It had been a jam-packed four weeks, but I had gotten some of my energy back, and everything was going as it was meant to go. I had made it through chemo and was about to take the next step. This major step. The one that would relieve me of my diseased boobs and give me new ones. Healthy ones. After that, I was determined it was all going to be smooth sailing. Everything was on track.

January had flown by, and my surgery date was just around the corner. I spent every moment I could trying to get the house and my life organized and ready for my recovery. I knew that was a lofty goal, but everything seemed like a lofty goal. I just wanted to do as much as I could ahead of time, so Kenny would have less to do while I was recuperating. It was going to be a lot for him, and I could tell he was concerned. He never said so, no matter how many times I asked him, but I knew he was.

All I needed to do was get to February 3rd. That was my surgery date. Then, I could finally take my foot off the gas and coast for a little while. But for now, I was in utilitarian mode. Checking off all the medical appointments on my list one by one. Watching the days pass on the calendar. Trying not to think about surgery. Instead, visualizing myself waking up in the hospital. The ice chips they would probably give me in ICU. Asking the nurse to get Kenny. I would want to see him right away. Then opening my eyes to see him looking down at me. Visualizing it all being over and finding myself on the other side. Visualizing the healing and recovery. Letting everything else go. *I was almost there.*

Mug Shots

Mortifying doesn't even do it justice. But on the other hand, very little should have seemed mortifying at that point. Over the past six months, so many people had seen me and touched me, and poked me, and prodded me. And I had long lost track of how many people had seen and felt my breasts. I was just doing as I was told, and going wherever I was told to go.

And where I was told to go in early January was to an appointment at the reconstruction surgeon's office. It was time to discuss my breast reconstruction surgery. This surgery would be performed in conjunction with my double mastectomy. And from the looks of my abdominal tissue (AKA: extra fat), I was a candidate for DIEP flap reconstruction surgery. That's where they use your own abdominal tissue to reconstruct your breasts. So, there was another silver lining in all of this — I would be getting a tummy tuck out of the deal. *Woohoo! I always wanted one of those.*

Kenny and I went to the appointment together. He sat in a chair just across from me in the exam room. Soon thereafter, the physician's assistant walked in carrying a 35mm Nikon camera and an iPad. I had no idea what was coming next. After a brief introduction and a review of the type of reconstruction surgery the doctor would be performing, the physician's assistant walked over and sat down next to me with the iPad. Then she began scrolling through a barrage of before and after photos of breasts, breasts, and more breasts.

"Here's another patient. This one is just six weeks post-op. And here's another one. You can see that there's minimal scarring. Here's another patient after six weeks. And this one is a patient after a revision surgery we did about ninety days after the reconstruction. Here's another one. And another…and another…and another. What do you think?"

"Oh my God, I think that's a lot of boobs, but they all look really good."

"Does your husband want to see?"

"No, that's OK, I'm fine right here," said Kenny.

"Don't be silly. Come over here and look at these boobs with me."

I don't think I've ever seen Kenny look more uncomfortable than he was in that moment. It was a lot to take in, but he and I were both pleasantly surprised by how natural the reconstructed breasts looked. This helped to put me at ease, because I really had no idea what I was going to be dealing with or what I would look like after surgery. I hadn't allowed myself to jump ahead to that part yet.

Then came the moment of truth. The physician's assistant handed me a plastic package and said, "I will step out so you can change into these. Then I will be back to take some before photos of you."

"What are these?"

Well, *these* were a matching set of humiliating pink paper garments that included a gown and ill-fitting undies. For my own dignity, I asked Kenny to step out of the room too. I didn't want him to see something he could never unsee.

I changed into this lovely getup, and the physician's assistant walked back into the room.

"OK, remove the gown and stand with your back against the wall."

"I feel like you are about to take my mug shot."

"It's not that bad, I promise. Just a few photos, and we'll be done."

"If you say so. Here goes nothing."

"Ok. Please look straight ahead. *Snap*. Turn to your left. *Snap*. Turn to your right. *Snap*. Now turn forty-five degrees to your right. *Snap*. And now forty-five degrees to your left. *Snap*. That's it. We're done."

"Thank God! Please tell me these photos will not be shared with future patients. Let's keep them our little secret. I don't want them included in your slideshow presentation."

"Not to worry. They won't be."

"Mostly, I am joking, but that was not fun."

"I know, but it's an important part of the process to take before and after photos."

"Fair enough."

. . .

Two days later, Kenny and I met with the reconstruction surgeon — who I will forever call an artist.

Make Mine a Double

From the beginning, I knew it was going to be a double mastectomy. Although I held out hope that I might be a candidate for a lumpectomy or a single mastectomy, something told me it was going to end up a double. Then once I tested positive for the BRCA1 gene mutation, the hoping game was over. It was confirmed right then and there — make mine a double. *No ifs, ands, or buts,* as my mom would say.

So, how do you prepare yourself for a double mastectomy? How do you say goodbye to your boobs? How do you mentally prepare for the surgical removal of your breasts? No matter how many ways I asked the question, I came up blank. For days, I kept staring at myself in the mirror. *Why did my boobs want to kill me?* I always appreciated them and treated them with the utmost respect. But, no matter how much I loved them, they had to go. *Why don't you love me back?* There was no way to comprehend it.

It felt like a loss of femininity. A loss of sexiness. A loss of sensation. *What would I look like and feel like?* I couldn't imagine it. My brain short-circuited when I tried to think about what the surgeons would be doing — surgically removing both of my breasts. And then somehow reconstructing new ones from my abdominal tissue. I had seen the photos, but they were all taken six weeks or so after surgery. *How would I look the first week or two? And how would I feel? How bad would the pain be?*

As usual, I stopped myself from thinking too far ahead. *Stay in the moment.* And this moment was just about saying goodbye to my breasts. Again, *how do I do that?* I asked myself that question so many times it was ridiculous.

Then, the day before surgery, I finally did it. Standing in the shower as the water gently fell over them, we said our goodbyes. It was short and sweet. One-way conversations usually are.

The Last Supper

It wasn't anything fancy, from anywhere fancy, but that wasn't the point. I just wanted a quiet meal with Kenny, Michael, and Joanne the night before my surgery. It just seemed like the thing to do. The perfect send-off. I dubbed it *The Last Supper*, mostly as a joke.

Michael was kind enough to host it at his house. I was craving a flatiron steak with horseradish sauce, couscous, and a side of broccoli. So, that's exactly what Michael ordered for me.

Everyone did their best to keep the conversation light and airy as we ate dinner together around Michael's dining room table. I wanted our time together to feel ordinary. No fuss. No stress. No talk about surgery. No talk about cancer. But we talked about it anyway. How could we not?

Then, I changed the subject.

"So, Michael, what's for dessert?"

"I ordered chocolate chip cookies for us, but they forgot to put them in the bag."

"Ah, too bad. I could really go for something chocolate right now."

"I can go back and get some if you want. I really don't mind."

"No. That's OK. I probably don't need them anyway."

That's when there was a knock at the door. After a couple of minutes, Michael returned to the table holding a bag.

"You won't believe this," Michael said. "It's a delivery from one of my clients, and it's chocolate!"

The timing was unbelievable. It felt more like a delivery from God.

Kenny and I left shortly after we devoured the chocolate. I was ready to get home. Ready to get my things together for the hospital. Ready to change my bed and clean my bathroom one more time. Ready to take a shower with the germ-killing soap as directed by my doctors. Lay out my clothes for the next morning. Set the alarm on my iPhone for 4:45 a.m.

Later that night, as I was lying there in my bed, I thought about the many conversations I had with Joanne about faith and God. All I could think about was my surgery, and I knew I would have trouble sleeping. There was just too much of everything floating around in my head. I needed to steady my thoughts. Calm my nerves. And then I remembered something she said to me a few weeks earlier. *Take all your stress, anxiety, and worry and imagine yourself packing it in a suitcase. Then hand that suitcase off to God.*

And that's exactly what I did. Just before nodding off to sleep, I imagined myself taking all the crap that was in my head and stuffing it into a suitcase: my stress, my anxiety, my fear, my worry. When I finished, the bag was so full it was hard to zip. I struggled and struggled with the zipper until it was finally closed tight. Then I stood the suitcase upright and rolled it across the floor into the waiting hand of God.

And God whispered, *I'll take it from here.*

Hospital

Just as I had pictured it, I woke up in ICU, was given some ice chips, and I promptly asked for Kenny. He appeared promptly, just the way I like it.

"How do you feel? Are you in pain?"

"Yes, but not my breasts. It's my abdomen that hurts."

"Well, I guess so. The incision was hip to hip."

"I know. I feel mostly numb up top."

"Yep, they said that's to be expected."

"How long was the surgery?"

"About 7 1/2 hours, which is pretty much what they told us."

"And everything was good? No problems?"

"Everything went perfect."

"Great! How much longer will I be in ICU?"

"Only a few more minutes. They are about to take you to your room."

Then I ran through my short list of people he was supposed to call when I got out of surgery. He assured me that all calls had been made.

Moments later, I was transported to my room, where I mostly fell in and out of sleep.

My hospital stay was just four days, and fairly uneventful. In fact, it was mostly a blur. Visitation was Kenny only, due to COVID-19 restrictions that were still in place. He came and went — mostly went — and I was OK with that because I was worried about Max and Stella. They weren't used to being home alone for long hours. And I was tired. Exhausted. You know how they do that thing in the hospital where they want you to rest, but then they wake you up every few minutes? Yeah, it was just like that. So, by the fourth day I was more than ready to go home.

I had been told to bring loose-fitting clothes. So, I had ordered several pairs of sweatpants from Amazon the weeks before. They were one size larger than my regular size. That should have been perfect, but the morning of my release from the hospital, those suckers wouldn't go all the way up. Not even close. I had underestimated how swollen my abdominal area would be, and my loose sweatpants were more like yoga pants.

I looked at Kenny, and neither of us knew what to do. Those were the only pants I had with me. Then my nurse walked into the room, and I explained the situation.

"They were so loose before my surgery, so I thought they would be fine. What should I do?"

"Maybe try cutting the waistband?"

"Good idea. Do you have some scissors?"

The nurse handed me a pair of scissors, and I cut small slits on the left and right side of the waistband. Still no use.

"So, are there some large scrubs you could loan me or that I could buy?"

"Let me see what I can find."

A couple of minutes later, the nurse walked back into the room carrying a giant pair of men's scrub pants. They were way too big, but I didn't care. I was just ready to put some pants on and get the hell out of there. I rolled up the bottom of each pant leg, climbed into the wheelchair, and off we went. *Problem solved.*

New Boobs. New Me.

Since my breast reconstruction surgery was done in conjunction with my double mastectomy, I never had to wake up without boobs. *Thank God!* That would have been too traumatic. Even so, I never looked at myself until after I was home from the hospital. And even then, I was scared to death of what I might see. I was worried I might not have the stomach for it. So, I had Kenny do it with me. I'm not sure what I was expecting, but in general, I was amazed. I still had a nice pair of boobs. Even though I was told that I would, and I had seen the many iPad boobs, I still had to see it to believe it.

And there they were. Not the ones I said goodbye to in the shower, but new boobs. They filled a bra, and that was alright with me. Everything looked and felt like it had all been moved around. Relocated. Stitched together. Even my belly button was slightly higher than it was before. That was fine with me, because everything that was done looked and felt natural. And that's what I wanted.

Luckily, I didn't have much breast pain. Most of my pain was concentrated on my abdominal area from the hip-to-hip incision. I was given pain medication, but I discontinued it a couple of days after I got home. I don't like taking pain medicine, and so warrior that I am, I switched to Tylenol.

I was told that this was a major surgery, so the recovery time would be about six weeks. I was also told I would probably regain some sensation in breasts. That's because they removed my nerves along with my abdominal tissue and reconnected them in my chest.

Even now as I write this, my body still doesn't look or feel exactly like my old one, but that's OK. Some parts are just different, and other parts are better. My breasts got a little lift, and the size and shape are indistinguishable from my old ones. As for my belly and waistline, I much prefer the new slimmer shape to the old one. It is much more flattering for my body type and size.

I like that all the parts came from me. They were just rearranged and reassembled. Glue and tape and scars. Visible ones and invisible ones.

Back Home

On my first day home, I realized I needed a few things. The first was a shower chair so I could sit while Kenny bathed me. I still had drains connected to some of the incision points, so showering became a two-person job. I always knew that day would come, but I pictured us as much older, and in my head, it was me bathing Kenny, not the other way around.

I also needed a couple of longer nightgowns, so I could easily attach my drains. Somehow, buying me new nightgowns became a job for Michael. I still have a hard time picturing it, but he went to Macy's and bought me some long flannel nightgowns. Likewise, Kenny went to Target and bought some granny panties for me. Yep, I needed those too.

As for food, it would be a few weeks before I was able to resume cooking duties. That meant relying on take-out, as Kenny's cooking repertoire remained very limited.

Doing the laundry wasn't exactly his thing, either. So, I would stand over him in the laundry room, directing his every move. *You can wash your jeans on warm with the towels. Wash all my stuff on cold. This can go into the dryer on a delicate cycle. This needs to hang dry.*

This needs to be washed by itself.

As for sleeping, my recliner became my bed for a few weeks following surgery. I learned how to sleep there on my back while clutching a pillow.

The doctors also wanted me to walk as much as I could around the house without overdoing it. I had to walk hunched over for a few weeks from the pain and tightness in my abdomen. That put additional strain on my back, which required the temporary help of a muscle relaxer.

Our bedroom was upstairs, and I was only supposed to climb the stairs once a day for the first week. So, when it was time, I gingerly walked up the stairs, one slow step at a time, with Kenny close behind. Everything got easier as the days went on, but I had to be careful not to push it.

CHAPTER 17: CANCER—FREE!

At long last, I find myself on the other side of tomorrow.

Anticipation

After my surgery, Kenny and I never talked about what my pathology report might say. I'm not even sure if he was thinking about it, and if he was, he kept it to himself, same as me. Was I afraid of jinxing it? Yep, pretty much. So, I kept it inside, waiting with bated breath. I prayed, as I often did, but without focusing my attention on that report. I just couldn't. At that point, I just had to believe it was in God's hands, and that was that.

Here's what I knew — the tumor had shrunk so much before my surgery that neither I nor my oncologist could feel it anymore. All indications were that my body had been very receptive to the chemo. So, going into surgery, everyone felt positive about my outcome.

Secondly, I had not one but both breasts removed, and hopefully, the only parts of me that remained were healthy. I had done everything possible to mitigate my current and future risk.

Still, I had to wait it out. There were eleven long days between my surgery and my appointment with my breast surgeon to go over the results of my pathology report. That's a long time to wait. I just kept thinking, *if they found something bad, they would have contacted me by now.* There was radio silence. *No news must be good news.*

Then finally, the appointment date rolled around. Again, Kenny and I didn't talk about it. Not on the drive over, and not as we walked into the medical building together. We just proceeded like everything was normal. Just a regularly scheduled post-op appointment. *It was anything but a regularly scheduled post-op appointment.*

When we arrived, the nurse escorted us into one of the exam rooms. We sat there, quietly waiting for that knock on the door from the breast surgeon. It was excruciating for me, but I never let on. We could hear a woman's voice coming from the next room.

"I think that's the doctor, so we must be next," I said, looking over at Kenny, trying to gauge his emotion.

There was nothing to gauge. He just sat there, moving his walking cane from his left hand to his right hand repeatedly, while looking down at the floor.

"Stop that! You're driving me crazy."

"Stop what?"

"Stop fiddling with your cane. The constant motion is all I can see."

"Sorry," he said, widening his eyes.

"Please, just sit there quietly. This is nerve-wracking enough as it is."

"Yes, ma'am."

"Seriously? I just need you to be still. Please."

"OK. I know you're anxious, and so am I."

He leaned his cane against the wall, and we waited in silence. I don't think it was more than ten minutes, but it felt like an eternity.

And then, *knock knock.*

CANCER-FREE!

There are certain moments you remember, and you remember them forever. They are etched like a tattoo right on your skin. You remember everything about them — where you were, the time of day, who was with you, how you felt, what you heard, what you were wearing, what you could see, smell, and taste.

Finding that lump in my right breast was certainly one of those moments. The somber look on the radiologist's face when she said, *I think it's cancer.* That was another. Then, receiving the call confirming my diagnosis. That makes the list too. But, hearing the words, *pathological complete response,* trumped them all.

There was no suspense to it. The breast surgeon walked into the room with a big grin on her face. She looked at me, looked at Kenny, and waved a stack of papers in the air.

"I have your pathology report, and the results show a pathological complete response."

"That's the first time I've heard that term. What does it mean?"

"It's the best possible outcome. It's exactly what we want. It means there was no residual invasive cancer in the tissue we removed during your surgery."

"So, I'm cancer-free?"

She walked over and put her arm around me, smiling from ear to ear.

"Yes! You are cancer-free!"

That's when I broke down. Every bit of pent-up emotion began to pour out of me. I didn't shed a single tear when I was diagnosed. I didn't shed a single tear while going through chemo. I didn't shed a single tear when I started to lose my hair. I didn't shed a single tear when I realized I needed to have a double mastectomy. But the moment I was told I was cancer-free, all the tears that hadn't yet been shed joined hands and made their way down my cheeks.

Cancer-free. CAAANNN-CCCERRR-FRRREEEE. I exhaled each syllable as slowly as my breath could release them. Letting the sound blow around my body. Encircling me with as much love and hope as the universe could bear.

It was Valentine's Day. It was the day my nightmare officially ended. At long last, I found myself on the other side of tomorrow. On the other side of the storm. It's what I'd been dreaming about for the last eight months. Finally, the healing was underway. And I understood the importance of staying grounded. Of staying right here. Feet firmly planted on the ground below. And I could breathe again. Really breathe.

The Lonely Wind

I was exactly where I wanted to be – away from the storm. The sun had finally begun to peek out from behind the dark clouds, and it was shining just for me.

A few years ago, I wrote a poem that speaks to this moment. I call it *The Lonely Wind*, and it goes like this:

> *Which direction*
> *Does the lonely wind blow?*
> *It is not east nor west,*
> *But to and fro.*
> *It cries out in a voice*
> *That only I can hear.*
> *It is quiet, so quiet*
> *I soften my ear.*
> *It wraps me up*
> *To keep me warm,*
> *And hurries me away,*
> *Away from the storm.*

Rest & Recovery

The six weeks following my surgery were a time of rest and recovery. My activities were limited, and I followed the doctors' orders to the letter – no lifting, straining, or doing anything too strenuous.

For the first couple of weeks, I kept it light and easy, mainly focusing on what I could do around the house. Short walks between the living room and the kitchen. Just enough to keep me somewhat active without overdoing it. Yes, there was pain, but far less than I had thought there would be. That was a blessing.

Sleeping was my biggest issue. I wasn't doing very much of that at night, so there were lots of daytime naps. By the third week, I was finally able to sleep in my bed. It turns out there's an art to propping yourself up into a comfortable position. It took a lot of pillows, but once I figured that out, all was good.

By the fourth week, I was given the green light to take short walks outside. At first, I only lasted about ten or fifteen minutes, but that steadily increased as the days went on. I was also told it was OK to lift five-pound weights, so I added that into my routine. It would be an uphill climb to get back to where I was before my diagnosis, but that was the goal, and I was ready to do the work.

At the same time, there was this marginal, yet palpable shift in my focus. I couldn't quite put my finger on it, but something was simmering in the background. I was caught somewhere between getting the best news ever, and knowing I would soon have to figure out what's next. Every time my thoughts turned in that direction, I forced myself to stop. *It's too soon. You must heal first. Give yourself time. No one is putting any pressure on you. Enjoy this moment.*

Creative Spark

Chemo brain was the ultimate creativity killer. It was sometimes impossible to even string a few common words together to form a simple sentence. And it was a straight-up assassin of my self-confidence. I was unable to write. Unable to create. Unable to do that which comes as naturally to me as breathing. Unable to have my thoughts connect in a meaningful way. Scared that *my gift* would never return. Scared that the voice that had been whispering in my ear since childhood had been silenced. I listened, and listened, but nothing came. It had been too quiet for far too long.

I felt like it had been forever since I had written anything good or important. Sometimes, a word would come to me, and I would quickly write it down to see if it might be the start of a poem, but then the well would run dry. Poetry can't be forced. It must come naturally from a sacred place when I am ready to receive it. So, all I could do was keep listening and waiting for the words. Waiting for that creative spark.

And then it happened.

When I least expected it, I heard that familiar voice. And I hurried to write down the words as they were delivered to me like a direct feed from above. The Devine gift of words as my pen moved across the page. I was starting to write again.

The first thing out of the gate was a poem. Not surprisingly, it was about my mom. It perfectly expresses the deep heartache I feel every day, and how I long to have her watch over me a little more.

Today my heart breaks
Just a little more
I can feel it in my chest
Deep inside my chest
There's a hollow hole
That can't be filled
And there's a pain
That just won't subside
And I cry
Just a little more
As I die just a little more
Missing you
Just a little more
Please, please, please
Watch over me
Just a little more

Double Stroke Roll

While recovering, I had more than my share of idol time. And for me, idol time breeds nervous energy, and nervous energy always needs a place to go.

The energy was trying to escape through my fingertips. I could feel the tingling in my hands. I kept catching myself wringing them and cracking my knuckles. And then there was the unconscious rhythmic tapping of my index fingers against my thumbs. Two taps on my right hand, followed by two taps on my left hand. Unknowingly, I just kept repeating the pattern.

Then one day, as I sat down at my desk to fill a little time, it became obvious. My drums were calling me to the throne. They were just behind me, waiting for me. So, I stood up, walked over, and sat behind my drum kit. I picked up a pair of drumsticks and reached across my body with my right arm to hit my hi-hat. *Nope.* Twisting my body proved too difficult without a bit of pain. *Not yet. It's too soon.*

When I stood back up, I saw the drum practice pad that I keep next to my desk. It's always there, mounted to a snare drum stand, for a time such as this. So, I grabbed a pair of drumsticks, sat down again at my desk, and pulled the stand towards me, positioning it between my legs. Then, I did what came naturally to me. I worked on my double stroke roll.

If you're not a drummer, you're probably wondering what the hell I'm talking about. Simply put, the double stroke roll is an alternating sticking pattern in which two strokes (hits) of the drum are played with one hand, followed by two strokes (hits) of the drum played with the other hand. *Right right, left left, right right, left left,* and so on. You just keep repeating the pattern. The idea is to play the double strokes evenly based on a particular tempo.

Practicing my double strokes provided the rhythm for my recovery. Slow and steady at first, and then gradually picking up speed. And the beauty of this exercise, is that with practice, there is progress. Authentic, measurable progress. And I needed some progress. So, I practiced my double strokes for hours a day, because I could. There wasn't anything else vying for my time or attention. I could challenge myself. Count the sixteenth notes. Create my own rhythm. Do what came naturally to me. It was easy to lose an entire afternoon, and I often did.

For as long as I've been playing drums, which is a little over a decade now, it's sometimes hard for me to say where writing ends and drumming begins. They both require rhythm, and each feeds the other. I've been known to write while sitting at my drum kit, and to bang on my drum pad while sitting at my desk. Both work their magic on my creative process in ways that are very different, yet very much the same.

Hair Growth = Personal Growth

I tracked my progress. Every Sunday, I would take four photos of my hair. One of the front, one of the back, one of the left side, and one of the right side. Then I compared the growth from week to week.

Before long, I began to see the parallel between hair growth and personal growth. With each passing week, I felt a little stronger. A little more like myself. The recovery and healing were becoming visible, and I was seeing what I needed to see. There was a twinkle returning to my eyes. My pale complexion was being replaced by rosy cheeks. The swelling in my abdomen was shrinking. It was all out there on display. Healthy cells had replaced the diseased ones.

At first, the hair growth was extremely slow. Almost undetectable. Then, miraculously, as if by its own instinct, my hair magically started to grow back into place. It didn't need persuasion; it just took up its old residency as if nothing had ever happened. Like it had been there the whole time. Each wild and crazy grey strand knew exactly where to go and what to do. *Muscle memory.*

At long last, my once bald head was again covered in hair. It was very short, curly, and mostly grey, but it was hair. Proving that my inner strength had indeed been triumphant against the worst kind of evil. You'd think I'd be really upset about a head full of grey hair. *Au contraire!* Grey was the new black, and I was embracing it. Every single shiny new strand of it.

Then it happened. By the end of April, I started to really see lots of new growth. Michael said it was growing as fast as a Chia

Pet, and he was right. The growth had really started to take shape, and I was elated. So elated, that I decided it was time for the big video reveal on Facebook. Time to remove the hat and share the growth.

I sat down at my desk, took a deep breath, and hit the record button on my iPhone. Another vulnerable moment caught on video. I was very used to those by now. But this one was also pivotal. That day, I didn't just remove my hat; I retired it.

Made It to May

May is a special month for me. It's both my birthday and wedding anniversary month. But there is something very magical beyond that. There's just something about May. I can breathe better, think better, create better, relax better, understand better. It splatters some mental clarity on pretty much everything in my life. It's like colors are bolder, and the only clouds are the big fluffy white ones. Even the sky is somehow bluer.

Each year as I turn that calendar page from April to May, I can feel my senses come alive. It signals new beginnings. And I feel ready for whatever it brings.

But this year, May took on a whole new meaning. It had been three months since my surgery, and almost a year since my diagnosis. It wasn't long ago that I wondered if I would ever see May again. So, making it to May was momentous. It was like May was shining a light on my future. I could see it. And I could bask in the unspoken promise of a life that is to be continued. It was a time of celebration.

When my birthday rolled around, we had a small family dinner at my favorite Italian restaurant. Afterwards, Kenny and I came home to eat my birthday cake, which I had made for myself. It was a yellow poppy seed layer cake with milk chocolate frosting. It was the exact cake my mom would have made for me if she had been here. So, it's the birthday cake that I will forever make for myself.

Since 2019, my birthdays have all come with another

undercurrent. The one that reminds me that I am facing another birthday without the woman who brought me into this world. That I live in a world that no longer belongs to her. I always thought my birthday was as much her day as it was mine. And now her absence has left a crater in my chest with nothing else to fill it.

Needing a Cry

It doesn't happen often, but when it does, it hits me like a ton of bricks. It was late, and I knew I should be sleeping. But I was all wound up and couldn't sleep. So, I decided to watch a TV show. From the description of this particular episode, I knew it was going to be a tearjerker, which is exactly what drew me in. I hit the play button on the remote and sunk a little deeper into the pillows on my bed.

Here's when it got me. There was a dream sequence, much like I have experienced myself many times, where one of the main characters flashed back to his childhood. It was the end of his life, and he was at home in bed with his family gathered around him. He never regained consciousness, but on the inside, he was wide awake. His life was beautifully portrayed by a series of flashing memories that spanned from childhood to old age.

Before I could even take a breath, the tears were streaming down my face. My eyes dancing between the TV screen and the photo of my mom that greets me each morning. I was thinking of her. Missing her. Thinking of myself and my own life. All my childhood memories rushing around me. My grandparents, aunts and uncles, and cousins. Holiday dinners and celebrations. Standing in Maw-Maw Pearl's kitchen as she made fried chicken. Flashes of me and Cheryl dancing around her bedroom as young teenagers, listening to Rod Stewart. Me and Michael sneaking around the kitchen together to steal a forbidden after-hours snack. Helping my mom bring the groceries in from the car. The hot Louisiana summers spent at the lake with my friends. Riding bikes and playing tennis. I was longing for the carefree innocence of the little girl I once was. Surrounded by the people who loved me.

I needed a cry, and this one was epic.

Surgery Number Two

Compared to my big surgery, this one almost felt like a footnote. In the long run, it was relatively minor. The plan was to have my ovaries and fallopian tubes removed about three months after my big surgery. This second surgery would be in conjunction with a small revision surgery to my breasts.

As per usual, I couldn't get my head around all the terminology being thrown at me about my breasts — revision of the bilateral reconstructed breast with liposuction and mastopexy, fat grafting, bilateral nipple reconstruction, etc. All I knew was that these things were necessary for making me whole again. So, that's all I needed to hear.

As for the removal of my ovaries and fallopian tubes, that would be done laparoscopically with just a few small incisions in my abdomen. The two surgeries together would only take a couple of hours, and I would be released from the hospital later that day. *Easy-peasy.*

Well, it turned out not to be so easy-peasy. When I woke up in PACU (post-anesthesia care unit), I was experiencing bradycardia. My heart rate kept dropping into the 40s. I felt very nauseous and out of it. There was an IV attached to my left arm, so I kept lifting up my right arm and moving it around to try and get my heart rate up. That helped, but only momentarily. Every time I stopped moving my arm and put it down, my heart rate would drop, and the IV machine would start beeping again. I kept repeating the exercise of moving my arm again and again, until finally the IV machine stopped beeping, and my heart rate was in the 60s. It took several minutes. There was a nurse in the room with us too. I'm not sure what she was doing. It all seemed chaotic. At the same time, I was having excruciating pain in my abdomen, and I was very tired.

I was also worried that I might be sent home that same day, but my doctors agreed that I needed to stay in the hospital overnight. I was relieved.

By morning, there was only minimal pain, my heart rate had stabilized, and I was ready to go home. So, with this second surgery behind me, I could now let the rest of the healing begin.

Do You Like My New Handbag?

New boobs are like new accessories. I have no shame or modesty when it comes to showing them to whoever needs to see them — mostly doctors. Although they are attached to me physically, I don't have the same emotional attachment to them as I did to my original pair. That would feel kind of like cheating on my old ones. So, when I take off my top, it doesn't feel like I'm revealing anything forbidden. It's like showing off a new handbag or piece of jewelry. At least, that's how it felt at first.

As time goes on, I have developed a growing fondness toward the new ones. The beautifully sculpted, nontoxic pair that are almost identical to the old ones. I've said it before, but my reconstruction surgeon was quite the artist.

Any fears I might have had about diminished femininity proved to be unfounded. My femininity wasn't lost; it was just reconstructed. Most days, I'm OK with that. Other days, it feels a little foreign. *Who is this person in the mirror?* Besides the new breasts, my hips are narrower, my waistline is trimmer, and my thighs are less full.

There are parts I miss, and parts I like better. It's about being comfortable with how you look and balancing that against how you feel on the inside. And not just accepting the changes, but embracing them.

Kintsugi

Kintsugi means *to join with gold*. It is the Japanese art of repairing broken pottery by mending it with lacquer that is mixed with powdered gold. It treats both the breakage and the repair as part of the history of an object. Together, the breakage and repair are said to make the object whole again. And although it is not the same as the original unflawed object, perhaps it is even better.

As a philosophy, Kintsugi is about embracing the beauty of human imperfections, rather than hiding them. It teaches us that all things — even broken things — have value and can be repaired. It's a good reminder that often true beauty is found in the cracks. So, just because something is broken or otherwise imperfect, doesn't mean it should be discarded or devalued. Instead, it should be revered and appreciated.

The gold fuses the perfect and imperfect parts together to make something much more interesting. In people, this is seen as an opportunity for personal renewal. Not just physically, but emotionally. And it's a reminder that we should highlight our flaws rather than hiding them.

I've thought about this a lot as it relates to my own flaws. They are on full display every day. I have scars to remind me of the war I have fought and won. Bits and pieces of me have been removed, relocated, replaced, and lifted. And I have my share of physical and emotional imperfections. The scars tattoo my skin with their pink hue, much like the lacquer mixed with gold. They are reminders of where I've been, who I once was, and who I've become. They are my battle scars. My healing wounds. My metals of honor. Still sensitive to the touch, but whole again.

CHAPTER 18: PROCESSING THE STORM

A life interrupted makes way for the next chapter.

Feeling Lost

My bounce back from my second surgery was fast. Within a couple of weeks, I was feeling good and was already lifting light weights. A couple of weeks after that, I was back on my Peloton. So, for the month of June, I mostly concentrated on my recovery and some semblance of a normal routine.

Somewhere out there was the finish line. I could almost see it in the distance. Scores of flags and onlookers waving me on. All I had to do was get through my last immunotherapy infusion at the end of August, get my port removed, and get my life back. It sounded so simple. Just three easy steps. I needed the closure. I longed for it. *Just keep moving towards that finish line. You're almost there. The hard part is over. You're cancer-free. Everything else is gravy.*

Physically, I was looking better and feeling better every day, but by the end of July, it all just hit me. Emotionally, things were still unsettled. It was difficult to articulate how I was feeling. I couldn't put my finger on it. I just kept asking myself the same questions repeatedly. *What was that? Why did this happen? Where does my life go from here? How long will I live? Will cancer come back?*

Then one morning, I walked into my office and sat down at my desk. Without even thinking, I picked up my journal and my favorite fountain pen, and I wrote in big bold letters:

I FEEL LOST!

I paused to look at the words. To really absorb them. To say them out loud. *Yes, this was it. I feel lost.* I had finally put into writing the crux of what I'd been feeling. *I feel lost.* I had been thinking that in such an abstract way for several weeks before writing the words. They had been sitting there on the tip of my tongue, waiting for their moment.

What does it mean to feel lost? I have felt that way so many times in my life, and it's difficult to put it into words. You just know it when you feel it, and you feel it when you know it.

This time it felt very different, because I didn't know what I should be doing. I didn't know what should come next. I was just aimlessly rolling from one day to the next.

I had fought my way to the other side of this enormous mountain. I had defeated the disease inside me. Everything else seemed so trivial. It was over, but it wasn't over. I was in this strange holding pattern. It was like purgatory. I was neither here nor there.

That's when I realized that everything that happened, had happened so fast, and I'd never stopped to process it. There was no time for that while I was in the trenches. But now, I needed to take the time to figure it all out. To put it in perspective. To get some closure. But I had no idea what that meant or what it would look like. I just knew I needed some time to reflect and process.

That night before bed, I told Kenny how I was feeling. Not a deep dive, because that's never a good idea before going to sleep.

"Hey, I need to tell you how I'm feeling."

"OK. How are you feeling?"

"I feel lost."

"In what way?"

"That's just it, I don't know. I just feel so lost and a little confused about everything that has happened. And it's all commingled with my grief over my mom, which I never fully processed either."

"So, what do you think you need to do?"

"I don't really know. I guess I need time to process all of this, and I have no idea what that means or how long it will take. I just need to try to understand everything that has happened and get some closure."

"That's understandable."

"I guess what I'm saying is that I need to do only this for right now. I'm not ready to go back to work or get a job or do anything else yet. Just this, whatever this is."

"And that's fine. You should take the time you need. I want you to do that. There's never been any pressure from me."

"I know, but I guess I feel a little guilty about not really working."

"Well, that's silly. I want you to take the time you need. We will figure everything else out. We always do."

In the days that followed, I felt frozen at best. Still not sure what I should be doing. I spent a lot of time sitting in my office, thinking that would help. Thinking the answers would just magically materialize. So, I parked myself in my desk chair and stared at the white brick wall of my neighbor's house, just outside my window. Counting the bricks. Squinting as the sunlight reflected back at me. Letting my eyes blur the image. Listening to the sound of life on the outside. Daydreaming. Meditating. Marinating. Ruminating. Allowing my thoughts to roam freely without destination.

Processing

At first, I thought I was *still* processing what happened, but I had never really processed it at all. Not any of it. I had been in fight mode the entire time. Doing what I had to do. Staying positive. Pushing myself forward and pushing my way through. But now, I needed to take a breath, to pause and reflect. It was up to me to figure out the way from here. No one was giving me any directions. No one was applying any pressure. This was all on me.

But how do I process this? I didn't even know where or how to begin. I just knew I had to break it down. Dissect it piece by piece. Examine every single element. And try to get some closure. I wasn't even sure if that would be possible, but I was willing to settle for a little bit of peace and clarity.

In just a matter of days, I went from *I feel lost*, to **WHAT THE HELL WAS THAT?** Chasing the answer to that question became the impetus for writing this book. And writing this book became the catalyst for processing everything that happened.

. . .

So, what the hell was that? I'm not even sure, and I'm the one who went through it. And as I stood there on the other side, I was certain there had to be something more. *But what?*

As it turns out, trauma breeds purpose. And I thought my purpose was to take my traumatic experience and use it to inspire others. Maybe in a small way, maybe in a big way. Only time will tell. The point was to pay it forward. To do for others, what others did for me.

So, I told myself, *this is not a time to be productive* — whatever *productive* is. It has always been hard for me to give in to those times when I'm not able to work. This was one of those times. And I had to somehow shift my mindset. To allow some space to open.

Part of me felt like I wanted or needed permission from someone. In a way, I was asking Kenny's permission the night I told him I felt lost. I was asking permission to take some time off and figure things out. But whatever permission I thought I needed, was unnecessary. Kenny was already onboard.

Drifting

For the month of August, drifting became a common theme for me. I could feel it. Kind of like I was being lightly pulled in several directions at once. There was no clear path before me, just tangled, meandering roads. *Where do I go from here? Where do I belong?* Cancer had been my singular focus for months, but now I was free. *So, why do I feel so trapped beneath the rubble? How do I climb out of the wreckage?*

I was starting to feel invisible. It was a feeling that wasn't unique to me or for me. But the difference this time was I didn't feel as *here* as I once was. I felt lighter. Like there was less of me somehow. So much less that I could just drift away if nothing was holding me down. I could easily slip away unnoticed.

There was also this inexplicable feeling of sadness, even though I had so much to be thankful for. I just didn't know there would be so much alone time on the other side of cancer. I didn't expect to feel so lonely.

Now that I was out of the woods, Kenny's focus had returned to work. That much I expected, and that's what needed to happen. But I didn't know what I should be doing with my time. I couldn't see the big picture. It was obscured. I have always worked towards something, but at that moment, I found myself in a holding pattern.

Borrowed Time

I couldn't help but wonder whether I was living on borrowed time. *Of course, I am.* Of course, we all are. But now, there was this new implication. A new worry that will probably never go away. *Is cancer coming back to get me, and if so, when?*

I felt like I needed to make the most of every minute before time ran out, but I had no clue how to do that. I was existing, not living, but I didn't know how to change that. I could literally close my eyes and see myself running against the clock. My thoughts would speed up to the point of anxiety. *I need to do something. Anything. What can I accomplish in the next five years or five days, or even five minutes? Hurry, before it's too late.*

My inner dialogue grew louder. There were so many things I could and should be doing, but I felt stuck. Unable to move. *Write a book, update my website, master my double strokes, clean out my closet, organize my office, go on an adventure, move to Louisiana, write it all down. Just get it all down. Ink onto paper. And leave a fucking mark!*

. . .

Facing your own mortality can really mess with you. But there's something empowering about it too. It is both an excuse and a justification for doing the things you never had time for or that you put off for whatever reason. *I almost died, so I'm doing this now.* It also creates a sense of urgency. A need to be more intentional with your time. It causes the pendulum to swing a little faster.

You begin to view time as a dwindling commodity. A recognition of your own impermanence. I felt it some days more than others. And when I felt it, the intensity was maddening. The anxiety spigot didn't want to shut itself off. Not even for a minute. It came out of nowhere and everywhere at the same time. Cornering me in all directions.

At the same time, I was grappling with feelings of irrelevance. My life was on hold, and there was this palpable feeling of disconnection. Disconnection from everything and everyone, including myself. *What's the meaning of life?* More importantly, *what's the meaning of my life? Have I lived it fully? Do I have regrets? Have there been enough adventures? Do I need a bucket list? Where do I fit in? Is life waiting for me? Waiting to give me a fresh start? A reset? Am I even relevant anymore? Have people forgotten me? Have I forgotten me? Hello. I'm still here.* I felt out of step with the whole planet.

Rocks and Stones

Ever since my mom's death, I often think about the Jewish tradition of placing a small rock or stone at the grave when visiting a loved one at the cemetery. It says, *I was here, I remember you.* As opposed to flowers, which are temporary and soon die, rocks and stones are permanent. So, placing a rock or stone at a grave is symbolic of the everlasting memory of a loved one. The ritual is a meaningful way of saying, *your memory lives on in me.* It is a tradition that is part of the act of remembrance.

I contrast that with my own feelings of impermanence, and I can't help but wonder who will visit me and for how many years after I die. Eventually, there will be no one left who remembers me, who loves me, who lights the *Yahrzeit* (memorial) candle for me. It only takes a few generations until people stop bringing you rocks and stones. At some point, my name will be spoken for the last time, and I will cease to be remembered. My memory will fade in the hearts of those who came after me.

Our memory on earth is as fleeting as our time. Nothing lasts forever.

I'm a Survivor

Life expectancy. This is a concept I just can't shake. And no one seems to want to discuss it with me. Not Kenny. Not Kendall. Not Michael. Not my doctors. No one. It's forbidden. Whenever I bring it up, the reaction is always the same. Whoever I am speaking to will just bow their head or look off in a different direction and tell me not to think about it. *Impossible.*

And people sometimes say the most inartful, insensitive things to you. Here's one that sticks with me from a well-meaning friend: *My mom was a fierce fighter just like you, but after twelve years and two recurrences, cancer finally got her.*

Don't get me wrong, I enjoy sharing my story. And I will gladly answer any questions, no matter how personal. And I appreciate when people share their stories with me. But when people want to talk recurrences and people who died, that's where I draw the line. In social situations, Kenny has learned to save me whenever he witnesses these conversations take a turn. He quickly changes the subject. It's just too much for me to handle.

Then there is the moment when somebody famous dies from cancer. For me, it was the death of Olivia Newton-John. I cried. Then I picked up my iPhone and downloaded several of her songs, and watched video clips of her from the movie *Grease.* I took her death very personally. On TV, I kept hearing the words, *after several bouts with breast cancer…,* and *after a long battle with breast cancer…,* and other similar phrases. I found myself wondering about my own fate. *Would cancer get me too one day?*

I'm now in this strange, exclusive club of *breast cancer survivors.* Living in a place the outside world doesn't fully understand. *Cancer survivor.* What does that even mean? I take it to mean anyone who has or has ever had cancer and is still alive. *Yep, that's me.*

One day, I decided to take a dive into Google to read up on the statistics. This is where things get dicey. It's that place I didn't want to go. That place I had forbidden myself from lurking. But I couldn't help myself. I sat there at my computer with my fingers firmly placed on the keyboard. I took a deep breath, then I typed the following into the Google search bar: *Survival rate for women with triple-negative breast cancer.* Then I quickly closed the lid to my MacBook. *Don't go there. Danger! Keep out!*

Still, I brought the subject up a few more times with my doctors. From what I have read and from what they have told me, of all the women diagnosed with breast cancer, only about 10-15 percent are triple-negative like me. And, it's an aggressive form of breast cancer, meaning it could expand and/or show up elsewhere in the body.

Now that I've had a double mastectomy and a pathological complete response, the likelihood of having breast cancer again is relatively low. But that's not to say it couldn't show up somewhere else. So, I have to remain diligent in the way I live my life, and with my regularly scheduled doctors' visits, scans, and so on.

As for survival rate, no one can really say for sure. My doctors have repeatedly referred to a 91 percent chance of a five-year survival rate. My understanding is that the risk of recurrence is higher during those first five years, then the risk goes down. Again, no one wants to talk about it, and doctors are reluctant to quote statistics, even when you press them.

Everyone keeps telling me not to get all hung up on numbers, but I can't help it. I want to do everything possible to stay healthy and know what my risks are, and survival rate is a big part of that.

The last time I tried talking with Kenny about it, he immediately shut me down. We were watching TV, and one of the characters on the show had just been diagnosed with breast cancer. Of course, she had the BRCA1 gene mutation, and the storyline was treating it like a death sentence. I could feel my throat tighten.

"Is this thing going to eventually come back and kill me?"

"What are you talking about? This is just a stupid TV show."

"Yeah, but I just keep thinking about how everyone talks in terms of the five-year survival rate. What the hell happens after that?"

"Nothing happens after that. You are going to be fine. Stop worrying yourself."

"I'm not worrying myself; I'm trying to understand the statistics and where I fit in."

"Don't even think about it. You need to let it go."

"Can't we just talk about it?"

"There's nothing to talk about. You're worrying about something that isn't even an issue."

That's how Kenny deals with things. Nothing is an issue until something is an issue. As you can guess, that's the exact opposite of how I deal with things. I need to talk things through, and sometimes, I need to talk them to death. But this time, he was right. I needed to let it go. I needed to remember that worrying would only invite negativity.

Feeling Stranded

Stranded, on the side of the road like a wounded soldier. A little dazed and confused. Trying to figure out how I got here and which way to go. Without the fight on the outside, people don't know or understand the battle I'm still fighting on the inside. The battle I might always be fighting. All the continued uncertainty. Truly not knowing what is around any corner.

My body has been through a significant trauma. That's the obvious trauma. But the other one. The one on the inside that no one sees and rarely asks about. That's the one that can really wreck you. And for me, it was all intertwined with the trauma of my mom's death. I was still dealing with that too. *It's not over. It will never be over.*

After all the positivity, I allowed myself to take a slight downward turn. It felt safe to do that now, as long as it was brief and didn't go too far below the surface. Just far enough to visit some of the what-ifs, and arrive at a place where I could begin again. Reload. Reset. Reboot. Find my way back to center.

From there, I would be ready to think about my next chapter, even if I didn't have a clue what that would be. And for the first time in many years, I didn't mind not knowing.

Then, one day, I found myself standing in front of the closet in my office. It is lined with shelves that house at least fifty notebooks and journals. Many have been retired, and others are waiting to be called up to active duty. Sometimes, I like to choose one at random and lose myself in the pages.

That day, I picked up a journal marked *July 2015* and began flipping through the pages. I'm not sure what I was looking for, maybe just a quick glimpse into the past. My eyes were drawn to one page in particular. It's funny how that works. The only words on the page were: *Michelle in transition.* I don't remember writing those words. I couldn't figure out the context. Chances are, I didn't even know the context in July of 2015. Sometimes I write down words and let them breathe on their own until later.

Inspired Inspiration

I think *inspiration* is one of the most powerful words in the English language. It is defined as the process of being mentally stimulated to do or feel something, especially to do something creative. I view inspiration as a two-way street; you get what you give. I think it's about pushing each other forward and motivating each other to do better and be more. It's a way of lifting each other up and exposing the best parts. It's about the warriors in front of me, as well as those behind. We are all links in this universal chain. Today it's me. Tomorrow it could be you. So, to inspire is to be inspired. Just knowing someone finds what I am doing inspiring, inspires me to do more, or at least to *keep moving.*

Inspiration is the one word that motivated me when I was at my lowest and needed it most. For me, it equals validation. It says I'm doing what I'm supposed to be doing, and above all else, that it matters. It's confirmation that I'm not alone. It's the realization that sharing everything I went through resonated with others and somehow helped them with their own struggles. This was a delicate responsibility, and I took it seriously. It also gave me the strength to fight my way down the healing path, no matter how rough the terrain or how far the distance.

Oftentimes, out of nowhere, I would receive a message or a voicemail from someone who was outside of my inner circle. The messages would typically begin with, *you don't know this, but I am so inspired by you.* To hear those words and to read those words told me I was fulfilling my purpose. I kept a notebook full of the messages I received. This was an idea that came from Kendall. She suggested I write them on sticky notes and put them on the wall of my office so they would always be around me. It was more my style to write them in a notebook, and to reread them as often as needed. So, that's what I did.

Several times, I received phone calls from friends from my hometown of Shreveport, Louisiana. I was blown away each time, because they were often dealing with their own health crises or personal struggles, yet they took the time to call and check on me. That made my heart smile. Those are the moments I will carry with me always and never take for granted. I think it inspires a little more kindness in me.

Through openly sharing my experience, and reading comments, messages, texts, cards, etc., I began to understand the value of the story I was telling. My attitude, positivity, strength, and message of *keep moving* was awakening a desire in others to do the same. That's what inspired inspiration is all about.

Sometimes we all feel broken, but trust me, there is strength — real strength — in allowing ourselves to heal while inspiring others along the way, without even knowing that we touched them at all. It's the most powerful gift imaginable.

CHAPTER 19: SAFE. HEALED. WHOLE.

I don't know if I'll ever achieve the inner peace I seek,
but that doesn't mean I should give in to the noise.

Meditation

For a long time, I had been in search of sustained peace. I needed it in every aspect of my life, at least for a little while. And so, I had to be careful not to let myself get drawn into any unnecessary drama or unrest. I had to continue to protect myself from negativity. Put up a protective barrier to keep myself safe. An iron dome to guard against any unwanted threats. I needed undisturbed stillness. I needed boring and calm. I needed some Zen. I was long overdue. So, I had to center myself.

Centering myself started with finding the right words. And the right words came to me in the form of a guided sleep meditation through my Peloton app. I had stumbled upon a specific meditation toward the end of my chemo treatment and began listening to it every night. It was a simple bedtime ritual that gave me so much hope. Everything I needed to hear was contained in the mantra repeated throughout the meditation: *You are safe. You are healed. You are whole.* These three concise sentences embodied everything I prayed for. Everything I wanted for my life. It was a meditative lullaby, gently rocking me to sleep.

I couldn't sleep without it. Each night I hit the play button on my iPhone in unison with my head hitting the pillow. Listening to the rhythm of my own breathing against the backdrop of the meditation. Focusing on my breath. Settling in. Letting my mind wander, then bringing it back to center. I listened and I focused, and until I drifted off.

You are safe. You are healed. You are whole. Safe. Healed. Whole.

. . .

So often at night, I have trouble sleeping. There are no discernible sounds other than the creaking of the house and the snoring of Kenny, Max, and Stella. I listen intently to the gravelly vibration of their breathing. So loud it drowns out the sounds of my own breath. Everything in my house is asleep except for me. I sit there. I lie there. I pray for morning. Lost in the quiet embrace of the night. So silent, I didn't even know if I was still there.

I often played my sleep meditation on repeat. I couldn't sleep, but I needed to hear those words over and over again. *Safe. Healed. Whole.* I needed to *be* those words. All three of those words. I needed to clear the path so littered with uncertainty.

Sometimes I would get out of bed, stand at my bedroom window, and peek through the blinds at the navy-blue sky, feeling tiny and insignificant in this giant universe. *Is anyone out there? Hello? God? Can you see me and hear my words?*

I began to bargain again, just as I had done in the days leading up to my diagnosis. *Dear God, please keep me safe, healed, and whole. My simple wish. My greatest prayer. Amen.*

Sea Change

One morning you wake up, and you realize your life is completely different. I think this happens multiple times throughout our lives. And each time feels like a defining moment because it is. I felt it that first morning when I woke up to the harsh reality that my mom was no longer there. Life was immediately different. The same was true the morning I received the call confirming my diagnosis. Everything was changed and changed forever.

But now, I am no longer in the deep slumber of the cancer nightmare. I've been tested. And through the grace of God, I seem to have passed the test. My faith renewed. So, I don't take anything for granted, and I never will again. I understand now that every day is a blessing, and there is so much to be thankful for. I have changed for the better. I have softened. I have a renewed sense of priorities.

One night, while on the phone with Joanne, I shared my

thoughts about how I was feeling.

"I can feel that there has been this change in me. I'm not even sure what it is, I just know everything is different now."

"Sweetheart, what you are experiencing is a sea change."

"It's funny you should call it a *sea change*. I've been thinking about those words lately, and they speak to what I'm going through."

"Oh Honey, yes! You have gone through a very difficult crisis, and you have come out on top, and you have done it in a way that most people are incapable of doing. You fought your way through and shared your story in the most remarkable way."

"Thank you so much! That's so sweet of you to say."

"Honey, I'm only telling you what's true. And you have been able to help others at the same time, which is just incredible. INCREDIBLE!"

"Well, as you know, that was important to me from the very beginning. And I know it will be important to how I live my life moving forward. I think it will help me heal from everything that has happened."

"Yes, it will. Like I said, this is your sea change."

"My sea change. I like the sound of that."

The Gift

Was having cancer a gift? I know some people say it was. I never saw it that way. Being saved and healed, that's the gift. The best gift of all — the gift of life. The gift of more years. The gift of more time. Knowing what my risk factors are and mitigating those risks, that's the gift. Discovering that I have the BRCA1 gene mutation, and that Kendall and Michael have it too, so they can mitigate their own risks. That's a gift.

Being able to share my journey was also a gift. And it was never just about me. It was always about helping others too, regardless of what they might be facing in their lives. The ability to share challenges, experiences, and grievances, especially from afar. To comfort and encourage each other. To offer prayers when needed. To share moments of joy, love, and healing.

Even as I write this — eighteen months after being told I am cancer-free — I am not fully healed. I may never be. But I don't regret what happened either. There's no point in having regrets about things you can't control. That much I've learned.

Lucky Bamboo

I bought a lucky bamboo plant for myself in May of 2021. It was an impulse buy right before Mother's Day. My mom had a thing for bamboo, so I bought it with her in mind.

Since bringing it home, the bamboo plant has lived on our kitchen table. I've never been much of a green thumb, so I didn't expect it to live very long. Against all odds, it's still alive today. This is the first time I've successfully taken care of a plant instead of killing it through neglect or overwatering. There's just something special about this one. There's an earthly connection.

Maybe it is the symbolism associated with the lucky bamboo. It is said to represent luck, happiness, prosperity, and health. It is also said to help with the movement of positive energy, promoting the flow of good vibes. Those are all things I want around me. And that's exactly what I see every day when I sit at that table.

I have since trimmed away some of the dead leaves and stems, but the bamboo plant is still very much alive and thriving. Yes, it's a little lopsided and flawed, but that's OK; I'm lopsided and flawed too. We all are. And that's more than OK. That's the whole damn point.

Staying Connected

When people run to your aid to support and encourage you, you can't help but feel loved and protected and safe. But, as soon as the risk has been downgraded, you feel that protective barrier begin to fall away. Then, once everyone thinks you're healed, they congratulate you and move on. They vanish just as quickly as they materialized when you were diagnosed. They don't realize they're doing it. It's completely unintentional. You no longer command the same level of attention, which is only fair. You can feel yourself getting smaller and smaller. No longer visible. Off the RADAR screen.

Yet, you still have this need for connection and community. You worry that everyone will forget about you, and that you will be left alone to battle whatever demons you still face in private.

But that's just it. You must do the hard work in private. You need the alone time. Healing is a solo act. It requires a certain degree of solitary confinement.

And yes, that's when loneliness can creep back in. And you might feel guilty for feeling anything other than blessed and grateful. But the loneliness is a natural part of the lingering trauma. It's a part of the residue that cancer leaves behind. Sink into it. Let it aid in your recovery. Let it shine a spotlight on your road to self-discovery and healing. And be open to where that path may lead.

Paying It Forward

I want to give back to the community that gave so much to me. To include myself in this far-reaching support system. To be a link in the chain for those who come after me. To pay it forward.

I remember all the questions I had after being diagnosed, and even more as I began chemo. They were the kind of questions that didn't rise to the level of requiring a medical answer. Just the kind of stuff you would ask a friend. *What kind of protein powder do you put in your smoothies? What should I bring to chemo with me? Do you wear a hat while sleeping to keep your head warm at night? Do you have a favorite meditation? How did you deal with chemo brain? How fast did your hair grow back after chemo? Can you recommend a good TV show to binge-watch?*

At first, I wasn't sure where to turn. The idea of joining a support group and talking to strangers didn't appeal to me. I'm more of a one-on-one kind of person. Fortunately, I had a few awesome friends who knew exactly what I was going through. Two were breast cancer survivors, and one was in the trenches right along with me. All three reached out to me within days of my diagnosis to offer help, comfort, and guidance. I had frequent calls with each of them, and even a handful of visits over coffee. Their insight was invaluable. And talking to them made me feel less alone.

So, as part of my own healing, I encouraged my friends to contact me if they or someone they know (God forbid) receives a cancer diagnosis and wants to talk. We all need a place to talk and ask questions. A place to give and receive advice. A place to offer tips and tricks for getting through chemo. A place to discuss shared experiences. A place to laugh. And a place to cry if needed.

I will be forever grateful to all those who supported me, answered my questions, shared their experiences, and were always available on the other end of the phone. And I am committed to always paying it forward.

Zen

Zen. What does it mean, and how do you achieve it?

That's just it. I don't think you just magically achieve it one day. It's about reaching a state of inner peace. A certain level of calm in the mind and of the being. Feeling OK about what has happened. That doesn't mean you have to fully understand it or know why it happened, but that you're able to accept it. A certain balance is needed, and acceptance evens the scales.

It's also about staying upbeat and positive amid a chaotic crisis. It's about having mindful awareness of the situation and refusing to let it break you. Staying grounded and centered as you power through some of the tougher moments. Finding the good within the clusters of evil. Looking for and finding silver linings. They are always there.

So, to find my Zen, I often leaned on my practice of meditation. Like exercise, it provided a little refuge. A respite from the tornado swirling around my life, lifting me off the ground. I found moments of Zen. And sometimes, moments were just enough. I learned to bask in them for as long or as short as they lasted. It gave my emotional and physical struggles a little air. It made them lighter, if only for a few minutes.

. . .

On the weekends, Kenny would often indulge me with slow walks through Houston's Memorial Park. It was an essential part of my healing and recovery. A little slice of Zen in a nature-rich setting. The sun and trees reflected in the water. The winding paths and trails filled with the sounds of laughing children and panting dogs. The crunching of the gravel with each step of my sneakers. It played like a soundtrack as we walked together hand-in-hand. Taking in the beauty. Breathing fresh air. Feeling alive.

CHAPTER 20: THE OFF-RAMP

Never stop climbing mountains. Never!

The Last Leg of The Journey

Before I knew it, the calendar had flipped to August, and I was nearing the end of my fifteen-month journey. I would have my last immunotherapy infusion on the 26th, then have my port removed a few weeks later, and then this whole nightmare would be done and dusted.

Have I mentioned yet that I need closure? *Yes, like a dozen times.* I can't help it. I'm just one of those people. Whether it's the end of a relationship or a bad situation, I need to know when it's over. In this case, no guesswork or analytical skills would be required. The final step would be the removal of my port – or so I thought – and that day was coming soon.

In typical fashion, I began counting down the days until my final immunotherapy infusion, and visualizing how it would feel to rid myself of the small protruding port, nestled just below my left collarbone. I would finally be done in a few short weeks. My last infusion. My last trip to the hospital. A minor in-office procedure. Just two boxes left to check.

The stage was set, and my feet were already racing towards the off-ramp.

Last Infusion

Finally, the day had arrived. I could feel the excitement as soon as my feet hit the floor when I got out of bed. And just as I had done so many times before, I hopped onto my Peloton to kickstart my last infusion day. Routine followed, and promise fulfilled.

The morning proved to be ordinary. The truth is, I wanted and needed it to be that way. I was feeling good. I had a full head of curly salt and pepper hair. I wasn't scared or nervous about anything. There was no bell to ring this time. *Just get it done. No need to make a fuss.*

I just needed to mark the day, but in a small way. Give thanks to the wonderful team of people in the Infusion Center, and then quietly leave. *Slip out the back, Jack.* This team had been with me for the last fourteen months, and now it was time to say goodbye. They had cared for me, held my hand, reassured me, comforted me, brought warm blankets and honey for my tea, made sure I had juice when I wanted juice, and crackers when I needed crackers. They even weighed me without saying the numbers out loud — not even once! They played an active role in saving me. They were the ones who administered the healing poison, and I loved them for it.

Bringing breakfast seemed like a gesture much too small, but it's what I did. I guess nothing says thank you for helping to save my life like bagels, cream cheese, muffins, and cinnamon rolls.

It was all over in a flash. Before I realized it, the infusion was done, and Kenny and I were heading towards the exit sign. I could feel my feet picking up the pace the closer we got to the door. Then it was a full sprint to the automatic doors standing between me and the outside of the hospital. Kenny was trailing closely behind.

As the doors opened, we were greeted by a beautiful day. Nothing but blue skies as far as the eyes could see. I paused and looked over my shoulder at Kenny.

"I want to shoot one last video of us leaving the hospital."

"Seriously? But it's so hot outside."

"It will be a quick one, I promise. Come stand next to me."

With the hospital behind us, I raised my iPhone to capture the moment.

"We are leaving the hospital. I am all done! Goodbye hospital. Goodbye."

Port Removal

Now that my infusions were over, I no longer needed my port. This was the last box to check. The final step to signify that my nightmare was finally over. My journey was coming to a screeching halt, and I was beyond ready. Beyond grateful. And beyond blessed.

I had two appointments that day. The first was with my oncologist for my ninety-day checkup, and the second was with my breast surgeon for my port removal. I decided that Kendall should be the one to go with me. I knew she would make it fun and bring the laughter, and that's precisely what the day called for. Closure was on its way. *Finally.*

When Kendall arrived at my house, I was giddy with excitement. I felt like a kid who had been promised a trip to the toy store after a doctor's appointment. Only, we wouldn't be going to the toy store; we would be going to In-N-Out Burger to feed my craving for a burger, fries, and a chocolate shake. I had earned every calorie.

So, I hurried Kendall out of the house and into my car. It was go time.

"Are you nervous about getting your port out?"

"No. Not at all. It can't happen fast enough."

"Yeah, I'm sure. I just didn't know if they said it would hurt or not."

"After everything I've already been through, I can't imagine this hurting very much. Besides, I'm kind of used to pain at this point."

"I know, and I hate that for you, but at least you will be all done after today."

"Yep. This day has been a long time coming, and I'm so ready."

"I know you are. You have been so strong considering everything you've had to go through, and I'm so proud of you."

"That means so much to me, but don't forget, you are every bit as strong as I am. Promise me that you will always remember that."

"I promise, Mom."

. . .

When my name was called at the oncologist's office, I asked Kendall to come with me into the exam room. Moments later, the doctor walked in. She greeted us with the same enthusiastic tone and friendly manner that I had come to love and appreciate.

"Hi! You must be Michelle's daughter."

"Yes. I'm Kendall, and I'm so happy to meet you."

"I'm so happy to meet you too. Can I give you a hug?"

"Yes, of course."

"You know, your mom was the absolute poster child for how to do chemo."

"I know. She's pretty awesome."

"Yes, she is. I was amazed by how she did everything so well and with such a positive attitude."

"Yes. Me too. Thank you for everything you did for her."

"You are welcome, but we worked together as a team, and your mom is quite the fighter."

"She sure is."

"Let me give her a quick exam, then y'all can be on your way."

. . .

The next stop was just one floor down at the breast surgeon's office. And again, when my name was called, Kendall came with me.

Less than five minutes later, the doctor walked in and introduced herself to Kendall. Everyone knew how anxious I was to get things going, so we kept the niceties to a minimum. I sat down on the reclining exam chair as the doctor put on her gloves.

It only took a few minutes, and I didn't feel any pain. The doctor used a local anesthetic, so all I could really feel was a slight tugging. When she was done, she asked me if I wanted to keep my port. Apparently, some patients like to keep them. *Nope, not me. I have plenty of breast cancer mementos.*

The doctor dropped the port in the trashcan and told me to take a couple of Tylenol when I got home for the pain. As for the stitches, she said they would dissolve on their own. I heard those words loud and clear. *The stitches would dissolve on their own.* And I thought, *and this whole cancer nightmare would dissolve right along with them.*

Kendall and I walked out of the doctor's office, and as the door closed behind us, I could feel a literal spring in my step.

"Come on. Skip with me," I said.

"Woman, you are crazy. You just had your port removed. You just got stitches. Aren't you sore?"

"No, I'm just happy. Take my hand and skip with me to the elevator."

"OK, woman."

And the two of us skipped down the hall, giggling like little girls. I needed the laugh. I needed the release. It was a moment to celebrate. To skip like no one's watching. And Kendall was the perfect person to be with me.

Later that night, as I sank into bed, I felt the relief of my port-free body. *I made it. I took the last step. My port is out. My cancer is gone. My hair is back. It's finally over.*

The On-ramp Is My Off-ramp

For the next few days, I was swept away by a wave of restlessness. I had this inexplicable feeling that something was still missing, but what? It didn't make sense. I had cleared the last hurdle. There was nothing left to do. Yet, I couldn't shake the feeling that I still needed an emotional off-ramp. Some sort of sign from above. A wink or a nod or a blown kiss. Just something that would give me the freedom to move forward. I didn't know what it would be; I just knew I would feel it — whatever *it* was.

And then it happened.

One week after my port was removed, Kenny had to undergo outpatient surgery on his rotator cuff. As soon as he was wheeled away from me in the hospital, I jumped in my car to go home and walk the dogs. When I pushed the ignition switch, I could almost see the world around me begin to illuminate. All my senses magnified at once. *What was this? What was happening?* Something more had ignited.

That's when I felt it. The sheer energy all around me. I was alone in my car. l was in the driver's seat. Punching the accelerator with my right foot. Gaining speed along the feeder road next to the freeway. Seeing the on-ramp in front of me, as a lump formed in my throat and my eyes began to water. These were happy tears, ushered in by those three words that fill my head, my heart, and my prayers: *safe, healed, whole.*

I was alive, very much alive. Pushing my foot, a little harder against the pedal as I made the slight left turn onto the on-ramp. My speed increasing. There was not another car in sight. Only me. Alone on the on-ramp, entering the freeway. Accelerating my way to freedom.

This feeling of pure euphoria rushing over me. My heart racing as my car launched me towards the sky like a rocket. Climbing higher and higher. The adrenaline pumping through my body. My fingers closing a little tighter around the steering wheel. Regaining control as I reached that moment of separation. I could feel it. I was separating from the cancer. It was explosive and exhilarating. All the weight leaving my shoulders. The weakness and uncertainty falling away from me and sprinkling itself on the ground below.

Smiling, as I began my slow, controlled descent. Reentering the earth's atmosphere once more. I didn't even need a parachute. I was enjoying the free fall. I could breathe, like really breathe for the first time since this whole saga began. I was in control. The last stitch had finally dissolved. I was safe, healed, and whole.

My meditation had manifested. My prayers had been answered. The voice deep inside of me said, *let that be enough. You've been given this chance, this opportunity, this reset, this blessing, this permission to live your life in a meaningful way. Take a breath and enjoy it.*

Be in the moment and let God lead you towards whatever is next. No stress. No pressure. No anxiety. Just take it all in. Breathe it all in. Steady your rhythm. Play in the pocket. Sustain that for a little while. Long enough to internalize the beat. Just stay right here. No one is forcing you to leave. Get comfortable. Take your shoes off. Slow and steady, slow and steady.

. . .

I go back to that miraculous day, that electrifying moment as often as necessary, and I remember the feeling as I raced up the on-ramp. Feeling the full release of everything inside me. Being set free in a moment of genuine clarity. There was electricity in my fingers as I gripped the steering wheel. *There is no going back. Keep moving forward with purpose. Drive yourself home.*

There is indeed life after cancer, and I felt it on that small stretch of freeway. Ah, the irony. The on-ramp was my off-ramp.

CHAPTER 21: LIFE AFTER CANCER

*In life you have to know where to put the comma,
and where to put the period.*

Victory Lap

It was time for a victory lap. I needed to celebrate. I had seen other people take these elaborate trips to Italy or Greece or France or some other fabulous place when they beat cancer. So, I thought I should do the same. But I didn't need an exotic destination, just a change of scenery. I yearned for specific scenery. I needed to go back home. I needed to feel my feet on Louisiana soil. I needed to sit beneath the twisted branches of a Magnolia tree. To see the marshy bayous and dip my soul in the familiar swampland.

It started with my strong desire to attend my 40th high school reunion in Shreveport. When the reunion was first announced, my initial thought was *no fucking way*. But, as the date grew closer and my hair began to grow, I knew I had to be there. But, it was a bad time for Kenny to take off from work.

That's when Michael stepped up and stepped in. He insisted that the two of us take off on a week-long pilgrimage through Louisiana. Just the two of us, and his Italian Greyhound, Louie. We wanted to make a nostalgic trip out of it. So, we spent time in Opelousas, Baton Rouge, Shreveport, Natchitoches, and all spots in between.

The emotional part was our time in Shreveport. We drove around and stopped at all our old haunts, including our two childhood homes. We both had a special fondness for our years in the second one. As I pulled my car up in front of the house, the two of us just sat there staring. I had done this very thing on every trip back to Shreveport since 1983, which was the year our family moved to Atlanta, before settling in Houston.

As we sat there, I reached for my iPhone to take a picture.

"No! Get out of the car. Let's go sit on the front porch and take a photo," said Michael.

"No, we can't do that. What if the owners are home?"

"It's fine. Come on."

"I don't know if that's a good idea."

"Let's go!"

We opened our car doors in unison and headed up the driveway.

"Let's at least ring the doorbell and see if anyone is home," I said.

Ring...Ring...

I leaned into the door to listen for the sound of footsteps from inside the house, but all was silent. I tried to peek through the narrow panes of glass on either side of the door, but I couldn't see anything.

So, we sat down together on the front porch, and reminisced and took photos. It was all so familiar. The red brick. The dark grey open shutters. The white painted railing across the long front porch. The iron railing on each side of the front steps. The brass doorknocker. The American flag gently waving in the breeze. It was a beautiful snapshot in time.

In a flash, I remembered what it was like on that front porch growing up. You could see everything from there. The cars passing by. Kids on bikes. Neighbors walking and jogging. The cute boys that lived next door. I remembered walking down the driveway and onto the sidewalk to meet Cheryl halfway between our houses. I remembered how happy I was every time I saw Maw-Maw Pearl's Fleetwood Cadillac pulling into our driveway. The stark contrast of her white hair and black rimmed sunglasses. Everything came flooding back.

I thought if we sat there long enough that our mom would eventually appear. This was her house. Everything about it was her. How could it belong to anyone else? She never wanted to leave, and as Michael and I sat there, I didn't want to leave either. I wanted to stay there. To go back. To be with her. I could feel her there. Hear her voice. Smell her perfume. For a brief moment, she was with us. Sitting between us on the top step of the front porch.

Then I snapped out of it. It was time to go. This house wasn't ours anymore. It belonged to someone else. And Mom was gone.

Michael had been right. We needed to sit on that front porch. We needed to feel it. We needed to hear our mom's voice calling us home.

. . .

Later that night was my high school reunion. I was overdressed in a sequined top, but I didn't care. I needed to sparkle. High school was one of the best times in my life, and I wanted to relive it for just one night, but minus the alcohol. I needed to be back home. To see my old friends. To hug as many necks as possible. To celebrate life. To make a toast to survival. To feel alive, and to sparkle.

Gravity

I get this feeling, especially at night. Long after Kenny has gone to sleep, and I get ready to shut everything down. It's always the same thing. I get out of the bed to set my iPhone and Apple Watch on their chargers and make that last trip to the bathroom for the night. As I stand up, I feel the gravity of everything that has happened. The pulling and tightness in my abdomen. The unnatural heaviness on my chest. The weight of it all just sits there, tightening its grasp. Reminding me that something very serious had indeed gone down. Reminding me just how close I came. How I danced around the water's edge. How I fought to keep my balance and not fall headfirst into the vast ocean. An ocean that didn't want me. An ocean that wasn't ready for me.

And for a second, I think, *my God what has happened?* Then I thank God for what has happened. *I am here. I am alive. I am cancer-free. I am blessed. I am at peace.*

Reminders

Will there ever be a day when I'm not thinking about cancer or being reminded of it? Definitely not. Reminders are everywhere. There's no escape. It always comes up at lunches and dinners with friends. It's on TV shows and movies and commercials. It relentlessly targets me. I'm its demographic. Reminders are there when I wake up in the morning and when I go to bed at night. Reminders are behind every door, just waiting to jump out and yell *boo*.

Every time I opened my closet door, I was blinded by the mere sight of my wig. Sitting there. Looking at me. Taunting me. It was impossible to avoid. It caused my hand to tense up every time I touched that sliding door. I dreaded pulling it open and the ensuing visceral reaction.

Then one day, I opened my closet door, saw that damn wig, and thought, *game over. Enough is enough. You're coming with me.* So, I picked up the Styrofoam head along with the wig, marched it down the hall, threw open the door to the guest room closet and said, *you live here now. Goodbye.* And that was the end of that.

Why did it take me so long to move the wig? I have no idea. Sometimes, the easiest solution is so obvious that we don't even see it.

Scars are another reminder. Although my body has healed, it has left me with scars. Physical reminders of what took place, as if I could ever forget. But the emotional scars are from the deepest cuts. The little incisions no one ever sees. The ones I'd rather not talk about.

"How are you doing," a friend will ask with a tilted head. "You look great, considering everything you've been through."

"Thank you? I feel great," I say, while the voice inside my head screams, *LIAR!*

I'm not great, but I don't have cancer, and that's good enough for me. Maybe I don't have to be great. Maybe I just need to ride quietly below the RADAR for a little while. Out of the spotlight. Fade into the scenery without drawing too much attention to myself.

Will I be looking over my shoulder for the rest of my life? No doubt about it! Always and forever. That's just part of the deal. Never get too comfortable or let your guard down. And always sleep with one eye open.

Routine Appointments

There will never be such a thing as a routine doctor's appointment ever again. I understand that and I accept it. Each appointment will forever be accompanied by my friends stress, fear, and anxiety. Just the general worry of what could be.

There's a hyperawareness around my health. It triggers my PTSD. Every pain, lump, and bump have my attention. *Is that just scar tissue or something else? Is that a new pain? And how can I properly examine myself when everything feels like a lump or a bump?* I call into question the slightest little cough. *How long have I had that cough? Is it allergies or something else?* I know now that anything is possible. And I never want to take anything for granted.

Even now as I write this, I continue to see my oncologist every ninety days, and have other regular check-ups, scans, and imaging. And this will continue until I reach the five-year mark of being cancer-free. Then, some of those appointments will become less frequent. Still, I realize there are always new developments in cancer care and prevention. New medications and recommendations get introduced, new protocols are observed, and additional proactive measures become part of the care. And that's fine with me. I've made it clear to my healthcare team that I am onboard for anything and everything that reduces my future risks.

Whenever I log onto my online patient portal, I see every appointment I have scheduled for the next two years. So many appointments, it makes my head spin. But I remind myself this isn't a choice; it's what must be.

Memory Loss

I am having some memory loss, and that's OK. There are just some things the brain doesn't want to remember. It's just too painful. So, you block things out, only to find them later. On the page or in a photo or in a video. It all comes flooding back as you close your eyes to sleep at night. Little fragments of memory. Slightly decomposed, but still recognizable.

Some of it is self-inflicted, because I don't want to remember. Because I choose to forget. Certain valves must be shut off and remain closed. It protects me from the parts that are too painful or unpleasant to think about. Too scary to commit to memory. Too real to exist.

Sometimes I catch that glimpse of myself in the mirror. That reminder of how different I look now. Grey hair. Newly formed lines on my face. A little older. I have been through the bowels of hell, and it shows. Yet, I remind myself that I took on a lot of incoming enemy fire and survived it all. That's the important part. The part worth remembering.

Maybe I'm not meant to recall every gory detail. Maybe it's like childbirth. Do you remember the pain of childbirth? I don't. That pain was quickly replaced by joy, and the joy is all that remains. I try to think about the aftermath of chemo and all the nasty side effects the same way. Just fleeting memories of the past.

So, don't allow yourself to commit the truly awful parts to memory. Just leave them in the moment. Be in the moment, and then let it go.

People Look At You Differently

People look at you differently. In a way, I feel like people have been looking at me differently my whole life. But since my illness, it has taken on a whole new meaning. It reminds me of how Max sometimes cocks his head when I speak to him. It's cute, and he wants to understand what I'm saying in his adorable way, but when a person does it to me, it makes me want to scream.

Even after cancer, I see it on people's faces. I see them staring at my grey hair and the new lines on my face. Then there's my breasts. They can't help but look there too. They can't help themselves. Are they wondering if I have implants or if I'm wearing a padded bra? Are they wondering what it looks like underneath? What it feels like? *Probably*. It makes me feel more self-conscious than ever. Sometimes, I also see this sadness in their eyes, like they're saying, *I'm sorry for your loss.*

Please don't look at me with sad eyes. I don't want to see the tiniest hint of pity. And for God's sake, please don't look at me as if I could fall into a million pieces at any moment. And don't hug me a little tighter. It says you could lose me. If you look at me differently, it tells me you see me differently. Yes, I look different, and I've been through hell, but I've come out on the other side. *It's still me. I'm right here.*

Life After Cancer

Sometimes, I think about all the things I wanted to do and thought I'd do after cancer. There was a list — a bucket list. But not surprisingly, not a single item on that list has been checked off. *A girl can dream though.*

Instead, my job from September 2022 to September 2023 has been to write this book. It's exactly what I needed to do. What I wanted to do. It's what I'd been doing all along before I even realized it. In a sense, it was my therapy. It allowed me to gain some clarity and perspective from a safe distance. To gather my thoughts and tell my story in hopes that others might benefit. Yes, it's about my cancer journey, but in a larger sense, it's about digging deep to overcome life's greatest challenges, whatever they might be. And how to do that with a positive attitude and a smile on your face. It's about reflecting the light that shines brightly on the inside. It's about staring down fear and anxiety and pushing through it, one day at a time.

It's OK if everyone else goes back to life as normal. To them, the risk is over, and so they assume you're OK. Their focus changes. Their priorities change. But for you, nothing feels like a return to normal. Normal has left the building, and you're not sure if it's ever coming back. And that's OK too. It's part of the process. You will find your own normal. Just give it time.

The important thing is that you have your life back. It's what you prayed for and dreamed about day after day and night after night. You have changed, and your body has been altered forever. And again, that's OK. There's no going back, only forward. So, keep moving. You might feel paralyzed – not sure where to go or where you fit in. But trust me, that's only temporary.

The good news — and of course, the best news — is that there is life after cancer. No need to bury the lead. Yes, it's different, but in many ways, it's exactly the same. I still wake up every morning in my bed, in my room, in my house, with Kenny, and look over at the photo of my mom. I get on my Peloton, lift weights, have a protein-rich breakfast, take a shower, get dressed, hang out in my office, read, write, play drums, walk the dogs, cook dinner, watch TV, talk on the phone, scroll through my iPhone, meditate, and go to sleep. Then, I wake up the next day and do it all over again. That might sound boring to you, but to me it's awesome.

AFTERWORD

Like any journey, there are left turns, right turns, times when you have to circle the block, climb uphill, coast downhill, take detours, drive over gravel, and encounter rough terrain. Sometimes it's a freshly paved road, and sometimes it's a street full of potholes. You might travel straight for miles or hit a roundabout and have to yield the right of way. Other times, you might veer off track onto dirt roads. You might be the driver, or the passenger, or find yourself alone in the backseat. You might rely on maps, navigation systems, or landmarks. You might get hot or get cold. You might roll the windows down, open the sunroof, or turn on the seat heater. You might hit dead-ends or encounter road construction. You might get a flat tire, overheat your engine, run out of gas, or have a blowout. You might have to get out and walk or push. But through it all, you must stay the course.

. . .

When I started writing this book, I wasn't sure what I would find. In many ways, that was the idea. It was much more than a cathartic exercise; it was a pilgrimage into the unknown, much like my cancer journey itself. An uncharted voyage deep inside my core to dissect all that had transpired. To see the forest and the trees. To figure out who I am today, who I was yesterday, and what my life looks like moving forward. To share the most intimate details of my personal, physical, and emotional well-being.

I was forced to relive a lot of memories, including some painful moments I'd much rather forget. But I was able to see things from a different perspective — a healthy one.

Even now, I'm not nearly as far removed as I'd like to be from the cancer or the trauma. I can't seem to shake it, no matter how hard I try.

Sometimes I feel like cancer is hiding out in my backseat,

225

waiting to jump out at me. Sometimes I think I can see him in my rearview mirror. I hate that he's still out there, but I can't seem to leave him by the side of the road. Trust me, I've tried. Oftentimes I've pulled my car over and yelled at him to *GET OUT*, but he ignores me every time.

Perhaps he just wants to watch me from a distance. Maybe he's just saying sorry. Maybe he's trying to make amends. Whatever the reason, he keeps me on my toes. Keeps me diligent. Keeps me aware. And I can live with that.

Meanwhile, I've had this time to think. To process. To reflect. To catch my breath. To see things from the other side. To ask questions and assign meaning – my meaning. To step outside of myself while going deeper at the same time. To forgive what has happened. To move forward from a place of peace. Healing, sacred peace.

. . .

I learned a lot about myself between finding a lump and finding my offramp. Innumerable lessons were sprinkled along my path. Some were specific to my cancer experience, while others were solid teachings about life and the way I want to live it moving forward. Many of those lessons were woven into the chapters of this book, including the lessons that were much more subtle. The ones I didn't even recognize until later. The ones that surprised me.

That's what reflection does for you. It gives you the space to look back without all the chaos. To revisit your experience from a place of peace. To see your own strength from a new perspective. And to decide who and what belongs in your life. Then and only then can you truly become healed.

ACKNOWLEDGMENTS

This book would not have been possible without the many friends, family members, and beautiful souls who loved, supported, and encouraged me throughout my journey. You know who you are! Because of you, I never felt like I was in this fight alone. You stood beside me — literally and figuratively — beating the drum for me and cheering me on every step of the way. Thank you so much for your unwavering kindness and generosity. I will never forget it, and I will be forever grateful.

ABOUT THE AUTHOR

Michelle Sandlin is an award-winning writer, author, poet, and breast cancer survivor. She is best known for her weekly *On the Move* column, which appeared in the Houston Chronicle from 2013 to 2020. As a columnist, Michelle wrote over 500 published articles. Her work has also been featured numerous times in Mobility Magazine, as well as The Houston Business Journal. Originally from Shreveport, Louisiana, Michelle studied Communication at LSU and later earned her BA in Journalism from the University of Houston. She currently lives in Houston with her husband, Kenny, and their English Bulldogs, Max and Stella. For more information, visit: www.MichelleSandlin.com